Making the Radiation Therapy Decision

Making
the
Radiation
Therapy Decision

by
David J. Brenner, Ph.D.,
and
Eric J. Hall, D.Sc.

Foreword by
Arthur C. Upton, M.D.,
Former Director,
United States National Cancer Institute

Lowell House
Los Angeles

Contemporary Books
Chicago

Requests for such permissions should be addressed to:

> Lowell House
> 2029 Century Park East, Suite 3290
> Los Angeles, CA 90067

Lowell House books can be purchased at special discounts when
ordered in bulk for premiums and special sales.
Contact Department TC at the address above.

Publisher: Jack Artenstein
Associate Publisher, Lowell House Adult: Bud Sperry
Managing Editor: Maria Magallanes
Text design: Robert S. Tinnon

Manufactured in the United States of America
10 9 8 7 6 5 4 3 2 1

Library of Congress Cataloging-in-Publication Data

Brenner, David J., 1953–
    Making the radiation therapy decision/by David J. Brenner and
Eric J. Hall
        p.   cm.
    Includes bibliographical references and index.
    ISBN 1-56565-333-5
        1. Cancer—Radiotherapy—Popular works.   I. Hall, Eric J.
II. Title.
RC271.R3B74   dc20   95-52097
                                                CIP

Contents

Foreword   Arthur C. Upton, M.D., Former Director,
United States National Cancer Institute   ix

Introduction   Peter B. Schiff, M.D., Ph.D., Chairman,
Department of Radiation Oncology,
Columbia Presbyterian Medical Center,
New York, New York
David J. Brenner, Ph.D., and
Eric J. Hall, D.Sc.   xi

Chapter 1   What Is Cancer?   1
What Cells Do Normally   1
What Cancerous Cells Do   2
Benign and Malignant Tumors   4
Different Types of Cancer   4
Metastases—The Spread of Cancer to Distant
Parts of the Body   5

Chapter 2   What Is Radiation?   9
Radiation and DNA   10
The Same as A-Bombs?   11
The Effects of Radiation
on Healthy Tissues   12
Doesn't Radiation Cause Cancer?   12
Doesn't Radiation Cause Genetic Effects?   13
Radiation and the Treatment of Cancer   14

Chapter 3   Your Cancer   15
                  The Initial Suspicion   15
                  Tests for Cancer   16
                  Facing Your Diagnosis   26

Chapter 4   Radiotherapy, Surgery, and
                  Chemotherapy   29
                  Radiation Therapy   30
                  Chemotherapy   39
                  Hormone Therapy   41
                  Cancer Surgery   42
                  Treating Aggressively—Curative and
                  Palliative Treatments   44

Chapter 5   The Radiotherapy Team   47

Chapter 6   The Most Common Cancers:
                  What Are Your Options?   53
                  Breast Cancer   53
                  Prostate Cancer   69
                  Lung Cancer   83
                  Cancers of the Cervix and
                  Endometrium   90
                  Cervical Cancer   90
                  Endometrial Cancer   98
                  Brain Tumors   102
                  Head and Neck Cancers   109
                  Cancer of the Larynx   109

Chapter 7   What Can I Expect *During* and
                  After My Radiotherapy?   119
                  Simulation   119
                  The Daily Treatment   122
                  Internal Radiotherapy or Brachytherapy   125
                  Possible Side Effects of Radiotherapy   130
                  When the Treatment Is Over   135

Chapter 8   Making the Radiotherapy Decision   137
Types of Oncologists   137
Choosing the Right Cancer
Treatment Center   140
Choosing the Right Radiation Oncologist   145
Finding Your Own Support Team   147
Talking with Your Radiation Oncologist   149
Weighing the Odds and
Making the Choice   150
Quality of Life   152
A Step-by-Step Approach to Making
the Radiotherapy Decision   153

Appendix A: Centers of Excellence for
Cancer Treatment   155

Appendix B: NCI-Designated Comprehensive
Cancer Centers   161

Appendix C: NCI-Designated Clinical
Cancer Centers   167

Appendix D: Where to Get More Information   171
Books   171
Videos   173
Other Sources of Information
About Cancer   173
Access to Information Through
the Computer   179

Glossary   181

Index   197

Foreword

Roughly one of every four Americans can expect to develop cancer at some time. Few, however, when confronted by the need to seek prompt and effective treatment of the disease, are adequately prepared to deal with the crisis. Naturally enough, few people know a great deal about cancer, and the ways it can be treated, which only compounds the many problems that people face in this predicament.

Although the search for a cure is a continuing quest, the real advances that have already come from recent research are not well known. In particular, there has been a major move in recent years to exploit differing combinations of surgery, chemotherapy, radiotherapy, and other modalities, depending upon the particular type and stage of the cancer in question.

Because some understanding of these matters can be crucial to cancer patients in coping with their illness and deciding on their treatment, this book should be invaluable to such patients. It should also be of great value to the families and other loved ones of cancer patients, all of whom are inevitably touched by the disease.

In a masterfully crafted series of clear and concise chapters written for the layman, the book explains the nature of cancer in its various manifestations, how it is diagnosed, how radiation, surgery, and chemotherapy are used to treat the different forms of the disease, possible side effects of radiotherapy, and the steps to be taken in attempting to decide whether to opt for radiotherapy or for some other type of treatment. By explaining radiotherapy's important place in the treatment of cancer, the book helps to dispel the widespread fear of radiation that can stand in the way of successful management of the disease. Finally, at the end of the book, the reader is provided with a helpful glossary and a useful listing of additional sources of information about cancer and cancer-related organizations, including various patient-support groups.

For the cancer patient whose survival involves a race against time, ready access to the information provided in this book may spell the difference between life and death. As a timely and reliable source of strategic guidance for cancer patients and their loved ones, the book fills an important need and should enjoy an increasingly large and appreciative readership.

ARTHUR C. UPTON, M.D.
Former Director,
United States National Cancer Institute

Introduction

So you've learned that you have cancer—many people's biggest fear. Not only do you have to get used to the idea of being a cancer patient, but the doctors want to start treating you right away.

More than half of all the people who are treated for cancer have radiotherapy as at least part of their treatment. When you first hear radiation being suggested, this can seem a frightening option. After everything you have heard about Chernobyl and Three Mile Island, they want you to lie under a machine and be deliberately exposed to radiation. How can radiation be causing cancers in other people, but curing yours? Isn't there something better?

The short answer is that, for many people, radiotherapy, alone or in combination with other treatments, does represent the best option—but certainly not in every case. This book takes you step by step through the many questions asked by people faced with the possibility of radiotherapy. Armed with the facts, you can make the best decision possible about whether radiotherapy is right for you.

This book is designed to help you acquire as much information as you need to assess your cancer therapy options in general and radiotherapy, in particular. Of course, gathering information is one thing, but using it wisely is another.

We strongly recommend that you share and discuss what you find with your physicians, and listen carefully to their views. All physicians are going to give you the best possible advice they can, but bear in mind the specialty of the physician with whom you are speaking. Whether they are surgeons, medical oncologists (chemotherapists), or radiation oncologists, they would hardly be human if they did not have some general inclination toward their own particular type of therapy.

Of course, as you will see, in many situations there is one obvious option, and every good physician will recommend that option. But, as you will also see, in many situations the choices are far less obvious, and it is here you need to be armed with as much information as possible.

We hope the information you get from reading this book will empower you, in collaboration with your physicians, to decide on the best treatment options for *you*.

PETER B. SCHIFF, M.D., Ph.D.,
Chairman,
Department of Radiation Oncology,
Columbia Presbyterian Medical Center,
New York, New York

DAVID J. BRENNER, Ph.D.

ERIC J. HALL, D.Sc.

Acknowledgments

The authors would very much like to thank their colleagues, both in patient care and in laboratory research, for it is in the cut and thrust of everyday debate that ideas are formed and experience gained.

We are greatly indebted to Peter Schiff, M.D., Ph.D., for correcting factual errors, providing much useful advice from his perspective as an experienced clinician, and for the preface. We are grateful to Eileen Rakovitch, M.D., and Nicholas Somers who provided many useful suggestions, as well as their perspectives as physician and layperson. The anatomical drawings by David Rosenzweig are gratefully acknowledged.

Finally, one of us (EJH) acknowledges the skill and dedication of the physicians, nurses, and technicians who cared for him while receiving radiation therapy for his own cancer. He salutes the fellow patients he met during the course of treatment. Their concerns and fears represent the questions to which this book provides some answers.

Chapter 1

What Is Cancer?

This book is about the use of radiation therapy in the treatment of cancer. So in this first chapter we will talk about the basics of cancer, in its many forms; in the next chapter we will talk about radiation—what it is and how it affects people.

Cancer is the generic name given to a group of several hundred different diseases. What do they have in common that prompts us to put them all together under one name? In order to see what is going wrong in cancerous cells, we need to first look at what happens in healthy cells.

What Cells Do Normally

One of the basic jobs of many cells in the body is to reproduce themselves to allow for growth or replacement of body parts. In any tissue or organ, cells quite routinely die, and when this happens other cells in that organ are programmed to divide and replicate themselves to produce replacement cells.

How does a cell know when and how to divide? The answer lies at the heart of the cell, which contains a tiny amount—less than one-trillionth of an ounce—of the chemical DNA (deoxyribonucleic acid). The DNA in the cell determines what kind of cell it is, where it should be, and what it should be doing—whether it is a liver cell, or a skin cell, and so on.

The structure of DNA has been known since Francis Crick and James Watson's great discovery in the early 1950s. Figure 1.1 represents a strand of DNA magnified about 10 million times. It consists of two spiral strands twisted around each other to form the famous "double helix." If we were to unwind the double helix, we would end up with something resembling a flat ladder in which the rungs and uprights are made of different organic chemicals. The four chemical "rungs" in DNA are arranged in different orders or codes, each carrying different instructions for that particular cell—a little like a complicated Morse code.

Contained in the DNA of each cell are instructions about how and when that particular cell should divide. This results in each tissue or organ in the body being of an appropriate size, and containing an appropriate number of cells, to perform its own unique function. For example, if a piece of skin is cut off, cells divide rapidly to replace it, but stop dividing once the damage is made good. If part of the liver is surgically removed, cells divide until the original size of the organ is restored, and then stop. Overall, the division of normal cells takes place under strict control, which is built into the DNA of each cell of every person.

What Cancerous Cells Do

A tumor occurs when something goes wrong with the control of the cell division process. Then cells can start dividing and multiplying without regard for their normal controls. Why this occurs is a question that has faced cancer researchers for many years, and we are just beginning to find out some of the answers. What we do know is the *effect* of cells that divide out of

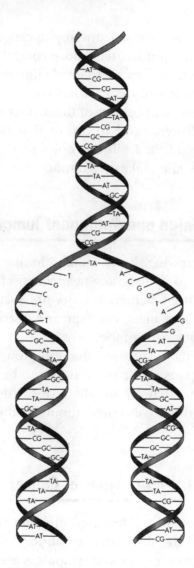

Figure 1.1 The double helix shape of the molecule DNA. The *GTCA* letters represent the "genetic code." The order of these letters determines all the inherited information about a person, as well as the information about what the particular cell containing that DNA actually does and when it should divide. The DNA is shown here in the process of replicating itself.

control. Supposing that just one rogue cell starts to divide without any of the normal regulatory controls, and suppose that its genetic instructions are to divide into two every day. So after one day, there will be a second copy of the rogue cell, after two days there will be four of them, after three days there will be eight of them, and so on. At that rate, after just a month there would be a billion copies of that original cell, which together would make up a tumor.

Benign and Malignant Tumors

A tumor that is growing slowly, remains localized in one place, and is not likely to damage any nearby critical organs, is said to be *benign*. Often benign tumors are just inconvenient lumps, although they may cause pain and discomfort by pressing on surrounding parts of the body.

On the other hand, a tumor that can grow rapidly, or can spread to other parts of the body, is said to be *malignant*. It is malignant tumors that are usually termed cancers, and it is these that we will be concerned about for the remainder of this book.

Different Types of Cancer

There are more than one hundred different types of cancer, and while they are all related to abnormal uncontrolled growth of cells, their causes and symptoms are often very different from each other.

For convenience, types of cancer are usually identified by the type of body tissue or by the body part from which the original rogue cell (or cells) developed. The major classifications are as follows:

- *Carcinoma* is the term used for a malignant tumor arising in cells whose main job is to provide a cover or lining of some sort to either an organ or a passageway. Sometimes these cells are external, such as the skin, and sometimes they are internal, such as the lining of the lung, stomach, or intestines.
- *Sarcoma* is a malignant tumor arising in connective tissues such as bone, muscle, or cartilage. Because we have connective tissues throughout our bodies, sarcomas can be located almost anywhere in the body.
- *Glioma* is a cancer of the brain, spinal cord, or nerves.
- *Lymphoma* is a malignant tumor of lymphatic tissue, such as the lymph nodes.
- *Leukemia* is the name used for a group of diseases affecting the blood-forming organs. It is sometimes called cancer of the blood, although it is actually a cancer of blood-forming organs, rather than blood itself. Unlike the other types of malignancy, there is usually no lump or hard mass involved in leukemia, but instead a large number of abnormal cells in the circulating blood crowd out the healthy normal cells.

Metastases—The Spread of Cancer to Distant Parts of the Body

As we have seen, the defining feature of a cancer is that it can grow rapidly, or has the potential to spread to other parts of the body. When a tumor has spread to a location that is physically separate from the original or primary tumor, this new separate part of the cancer is called a metastasis. Basically, there are three ways in which a malignant tumor can spread.

The first way in which a tumor can spread is simply that the primary tumor continues to grow larger. All cells, including tumor cells, need some amount of nutrients to survive, and tumors develop their own system of blood vessels. These veins and arteries allow blood to flow through the tumor, provide the tumor cells with oxygen, and so allow them to continue growing.

This blood flow near or through the tumor provides the second way in which a cancer can spread. Tumor cells can grow through the walls of the nearby blood vessels and get carried along as the blood flows. They can then end up settling in some distant part of the body where, if the conditions are right, they may start growing again.

The third route for cancer cells to spread is via the body's lymphatic system. This is a series of thin vessels that run throughout the body. Circulating through this system is a liquid (lymph) whose job is to carry off and drain away toxic and infectious materials from all over the body. At various locations, the lymphatic system has lymph nodes, bean- or spherical-shaped receptacles into which the waste material is drained. We have lymph nodes throughout our body, such as under our armpits, behind our knees, and in the groin. For example, the familiar "swollen glands" during a viral throat infection result from the buildup of waste material in lymph nodes in the neck. Because the lymph node system is designed to deal with extra waste products, tumor cells have a tendency to spread to the lymph nodes. Once they are there, they tend to grow into a hard lump, and have the potential to spread to other parts of the body through the lymphatic system.

How Could It Happen to Me?

Once anyone has been diagnosed with cancer, an obvious first thought is "why me?" The fact is, however, that with only a few exceptions, we simply cannot say what is the cause of any particular cancer.

Some rare types of cancers are clearly inherited. One example is retinoblastoma, a cancer of the retina. Another example is Wilm's tumor, a cancer of the kidney. These inherited cancers tend to occur early in life, particularly in children.

More commonly, some cancers have a partial hereditary component—in other words, some or all of the members of a particular family may be more likely than average to develop a particular cancer. For example, if a woman has several family members who have had breast cancer, she is more likely to get breast cancer herself. On the other hand, many—and probably most—cancers do not seem to show any hereditary factors at all.

Within the last few years, scientific advances have resulted in the identification of parts of DNA, called genes, which can predispose some people to some kinds of cancer. One of the first to be identified was the gene involved in the inherited form of colon cancer, and soon after that the genes involved in some (relatively rare) forms of breast cancer. This is a rapidly advancing field and it is possible that within a few years the genes involved in many common types of cancer will be identified.

At present, however, it appears that most cancers are not associated with hereditary genes—some internal personal factor making certain people especially susceptible. If the cause of most cancers is not something inside our DNA, then it would seem reasonable to assume that these cancers must be related to our environment. And indeed some types of pollution have been clearly linked to cancer. The most obvious example is the link between tobacco smoke and lung cancer. Until smoking became common in the last fifty years, lung cancer was quite a rare disease. Other cancers have been linked with high exposures to different pollutants, such as asbestos, pesticides and, as we have seen, X rays.

But most people who develop cancer don't smoke and have

not been exposed to high levels of these pollutants. So why are they getting cancer? And why are cancer rates on the increase?

One factor that has led to an increase in the number of people developing cancer is the enormous advances that have been made in other fields of medicine. We are living much longer than we did a hundred years ago, mainly because we can control infectious diseases with antibiotics. Thus we have more and more years during which to develop cancer—the longer we live, the higher our chances of developing cancer.

The bottom line is that, except in a few cases, it is impossible to give a reason as to why any particular individual developed cancer. The exception is lung cancer in smokers. Other than that, while each cancer surely does have one or more causes, we do not yet know enough to say what those causes are.

In this chapter, we have talked about cancer in its many forms. Now we turn to radiation. In the next chapter we talk about what radiation is and how it affects people. Then, throughout the rest of this book, we will talk about how radiation is used to treat cancer.

Chapter 2

What Is Radiation?

More than half of all people who are treated for cancer have radiation therapy as part of their treatment. The idea of radiation often brings out strong emotions in people. Thoughts of atomic bombs, and the accidents at the Three Mile Island and Chernobyl nuclear power plants, often spring to mind, and are hardly reassuring. In reality, radiation is a lot less mysterious. In this chapter we will talk about what radiation is, and how exactly it affects us.

Our knowledge about radiation is just a century old. X rays were first discovered by Wilhelm Roentgen in 1895, and just a year later they were being used to examine fractured bones. In fact, there are many different types of radiation: alpha rays, gamma rays, beta rays, neutrons, radio waves, X rays, and light waves, to name but a few. For our purposes, however, we mainly need to consider the type discovered by Roentgen: X rays.

X rays are invisible, fast-moving packets of energy, moving just like light rays, at the speed of light. In fact there is no fundamental difference between X rays and light rays; the only difference is that X rays are more energetic. Occasionally you will also hear talk of *gamma rays*, as well as X rays. For our purposes here, there is no major difference between X and gamma rays. External radiotherapy (see Chapter 4) is usually given with X rays, while internal radiotherapy (see Chapter 4) is usually given with gamma rays. In terms of their curative effects in radiotherapy, there is no difference between them.

The fact that X and gamma rays are both very energetic is crucial to their use in radiotherapy. If X rays are aimed at living tissue, they have enough energy to "knock out" some of the electrons whose job it is to hold together the molecules in the living tissue. This process of knocking out electrons is similar to two billiard balls colliding: the X ray is the cue ball, and when it hits the target ball—an electron—it knocks the electron away from its correct location.

This process of knocking out electrons is usually called *ionization*. Radiations, like X or gamma rays, that can cause ionization are far more biologically hazardous than lower-energy radiations like light rays, which cannot ionize.

Radiation and DNA

The most common molecule in the human body is water (H_2O), which consists of two hydrogen atoms and one oxygen atom held together with electrons. From a biological point of view, however, the most important molecule in the body is larger and more complicated: DNA (deoxyribonucleic acid). As we saw in Chapter 1, DNA plays a central role in life itself, as it is the molecule controlling cell division and replication. Let's talk about what can happen if DNA is hit by X rays.

The DNA molecule consists of many atoms arranged in two spiral strands—the famous "double helix"(see Fig. 1.1). As with all molecules, the atoms in this structure are held in their correct place by electrons. When X rays pass through DNA, they can knock out some of these electrons, causing breaks or distortions in the DNA's spiral shape. In general, the body is very efficient about mending this sort of damage. Chemicals called enzymes will quickly arrive at the scene and cut out the damaged piece. Then they will make a replacement piece of DNA, put it in position, and glue the ends back together again—a remarkable achievement!

While these repair systems for fixing damaged DNA are extraordinarily good, they are not perfect. Particularly at the high doses of radiation aimed at a cancer during radiotherapy, some of the DNA damage may not be repaired correctly—or even at all. What can happen then?

The most common result when the DNA is not perfectly repaired is that it loses its ability to guide the cell through the process of division or replication. When this happens, the cell loses its ability to divide and, practically speaking, can be considered dead. Of course, if that cell were a cancer cell, this is exactly the result we want—the cell can no longer divide in an uncontrolled way.

The Same as A-Bombs?

The last section described the basic rationale for radiotherapy—the ability of X or gamma rays to damage DNA and so prevent cancer cells from dividing.

Of course, radiation has not always been used for such good reasons. The terrible biological damage to the victims of the atomic bombs at Hiroshima and Nagasaki was caused by radiation through the same processes that stop cancer cells from dividing after radiotherapy. The big difference, though, is that the entire bodies of the unfortunate victims of the atomic bombs received a high dose of radiation. Because some body organs, like the gut and the blood-forming organs, function by constant cell division, these organs cannot tolerate exposure to a high dose of radiation. The fundamental difference in radiotherapy is that the radiation is usually targeted only toward the cancer, and not the entire body.

The Effects of Radiation on Healthy Tissues

The prime goal of radiotherapy is to deliver as much radiation as possible to the cancer and as little as possible to normal tissues. A perfect treatment, however, where the healthy, normal tissues receive *no* radiation, is currently not possible, and probably never will be. So it is an unfortunate but inevitable fact that some healthy tissues will also be damaged during radiotherapy, and this damage will translate itself into some side effects. More and more, radiotherapy technology is being improved so that fewer normal tissue cells—or more cancer cells—will be damaged. We'll learn more about that in Chapter 4.

Ultimately, as we will discuss in Chapter 8, the question of side effects in radiotherapy boils down to asking "What is the risk relative to the potential benefits?" All possible treatments have risks and benefits associated with them, and our aim here is to enable you to weigh the odds in as informed a way as possible.

Doesn't Radiation Cause Cancer?

The short answer is that radiation can cause cancer. The way it causes cancer is similar to the way in which it can stop cells from dividing. As we have seen, when radiation damages DNA by knocking out electrons, the body's defense mechanisms step in to repair the damage. Once in a great while, although the damage is repaired sufficiently well that the cell is able to divide, the cell's instructions, telling it when and how to divide, end up being damaged. (Recall that all these instructions are coded in the DNA itself.)

So now we could have a situation where cells are dividing, but their controls telling them when and how to divide are damaged. This is exactly what cancer is. It is important to realize, however, that radiation cannot *immediately* cause cancer. On average, even on those rare occasions when exposure to radiation does cause cancer, the time between radiation exposure and the cancer appearing is very long—usually more than twenty years.

In fact, we know quite a lot about the risks of radiation producing cancer, mostly because of the tragic events at Hiroshima and Nagasaki. We certainly know more about the risks of radiation-induced cancer than we do about the risks of cancer from chemicals, such as chemotherapy agents, and the fact is the risks are extremely small.

Doesn't Radiation Cause Genetic Effects?

A genetic effect is biological damage that can be inherited, meaning it can be passed on to offspring. The short answer is probably yes, radiation does cause genetic effects, but the risks are minute. In fact, over the past fifty years, there has been an enormous effort to study the roughly 70,000 children of survivors of the atomic bombings at Hiroshima and Nagasaki. To date, no evidence has been found of any health effects caused by the radiation exposure to their parents.

On the other hand, studies of animals exposed to radiation do show that radiation damage can, in principle, be passed on to subsequent generations, if the reproductive organs get a sufficiently high dose of radiation. But the risk in the context of radiotherapy is extremely small.

A more relevant issue concerns the rare occasions when a

relatively young person develops a cancer either in or very near the reproductive organs—the ovaries or the testes. In these situations, radiation therapy may well affect that person's fertility—the ability to conceive or reproduce children.

Radiation and the Treatment of Cancer

As we saw, X rays were discovered in 1895 by Wilhelm Roentgen. Within a couple of years it was realized that radiation could damage human tissue. In fact, some of the earliest experiments were conducted by Marie Curie's husband, Pierre Curie, who put some radioactive material on his arm and observed a radiation "burn." By the beginning of the twentieth century, many scientists, realizing that radiation could damage human tissues, were experimenting by treating cancer with radiation. By 1900, the first "cure" had been reported.

By the 1930s the basic biological principles of treating human cancers with radiation had been worked out. The major developments in radiation therapy since then have largely been in the technology used for treatments—more sophisticated machines and, of course, the advent of computers.

In later chapters we focus on how radiation is currently used for treating different cancers. But first, in the next chapter, we talk about how cancers are diagnosed.

Chapter 3

Your Cancer

There are more than one hundred different cancers, and for each one, many different subcategories. Perhaps *the* most critical information you and your physicians will need in order to arrive at your best treatment option is the exact details of your cancer. This chapter is about the process of finding out these details—the process of cancer diagnosis.

The Initial Suspicion

Probably the most important rule in the whole field of cancer is *the earlier the cancer is diagnosed, the better the likely outcome.* So regular routine physical checkups are crucial.

There are a few special tests for specific types of cancer, such as mammograms for breast cancer, the Pap smear test for cervical cancer, and the PSA prostate test. The great advantage of these tests is that they can potentially catch the cancer early, before any physical symptoms appear. So these tests are an extremely good idea for individuals in the recommended age groups.

In many cases, however, it is the patient who detects the first sign of cancer. The American Cancer Society describes seven early warning signals for cancer:

- change in bowel or bladder habits
- a sore that does not heal
- unusual bleeding or discharge
- thickening or lump in the breast or any other part of the body
- indigestion or difficulty swallowing
- obvious change in a wart or mole
- nagging cough or hoarseness

Everyone should be aware of these, and take them seriously.

Tests for Cancer

Once there is a suspicion of cancer, the next step is more detailed tests that will show clearly whether you have cancer. The particular types of tests you will have will depend on the location of the suspected cancer, but generally the tests fall into two basic categories:

- imaging tests, where the physician attempts to "see" the cancer, either directly or indirectly
- direct examination of samples of tissue or blood

Let's look at these types of tests in a little more detail.

Imaging Tests

"Seeing" the cancer does not always mean viewing it directly by eye. Often the cancer is viewed indirectly, with the aid of various high-tech imaging devices. The most common types of cancer imaging techniques are:

- X rays
- CT (computerized tomography) scans
- MRI (magnetic resonance imaging)
- nuclear medicine scans
- ultrasound
- endoscopy

The most common imaging technique, and often the first one used, is the *X ray*. Here, a stream of X rays is aimed in the direction of the suspected region, and a picture is taken on an X-ray film located on the far side of the body. A tumor often shows up as a dark shadow or an unusual distortion of the organs, and can be spotted by an experienced radiologist.

Sometimes, depending on the size and location of the possible cancer, its X-ray shadow is not visible on the film. One solution is to use a "contrast agent" in the region of the suspected tumor, which will allow greater contrast between the tumor shadow and the surrounding region. These contrast agents are most commonly used in the bowel region (the barium enema), the stomach (the barium "meal"), and the kidney.

CT (computerized tomography) scans are really just sophisticated high-tech X-ray scans. A conventional X-ray picture consists of only a shadow on an X-ray film, so the radiologist can get an idea of the height and width of the possible tumor, but only limited information about its depth. In other words, just like any other shadow, it is a two-dimensional image. Essentially a CT scan involves taking pictures of the tumor from various positions. These pictures are then combined, using a computer, to produce a three-dimensional picture. This gives a much better idea of the size and shape of the tumor and the surrounding healthy tissues—something that will be very important when it comes to considering treatment options.

Although three-dimensional scans are most often done

using X rays, they are increasingly being performed with *MRI* (*magnetic resonance imaging*). Just like X-ray CT, an MRI scan produces a three-dimensional picture of the tumor. It does not use X rays to produce the images, however; instead it uses an extremely powerful magnet that produces a tiny change in all the atoms in the body—an effect that goes away when the magnet is turned off. Different elements in the body, such as hydrogen, are affected differently by the powerful magnet, and these differences can be used to make a "map" or image of all the hydrogen in the suspect region of the body, which in turn can be used to produce a three-dimensional image of the tumor.

In fact, the X-ray CT and the MRI produce slightly different types of pictures, which are highly complementary to each other. Both techniques are often used to get different images of the same suspect site.

Nuclear medicine is often described as taking an X-ray picture in reverse. With conventional X rays, the source of radiation—the X-ray machine—is outside the body, and the X rays are aimed from there at the tumor. In nuclear medicine, on the other hand, the idea is to put the source of the radiation actually inside the tumor and to detect the rays when they exit the body. A computer can then use that information to produce an image of where the X rays started from—that is, the tumor. As an example, the thyroid is very efficient at taking up iodine, so ingesting radioactive iodine (in other words, iodine that emits radiation) will produce a source of radiation that starts from inside the thyroid. Detecting this radiation when it emerges from the body allows a computer to estimate the shape of the thyroid.

Another option is *ultrasound*. This is just like the "sonar" you hear in submarines or movies about submarines. What happens is a high-frequency sound wave is bounced off the target—in this case your body. This sound wave will bounce off different organs—or a tumor—in slightly different ways. A microphone picks up the reflected sound waves, again enabling a computer to produce a picture of the region at which the ultrasound was aimed. Ultrasound is most familiar as a way of examining the fetus during pregnancy, but it is often used to search for possible tumors.

All the imaging techniques that we have looked at so far are "indirect"—something is bounced off or passed through the suspicious region, and the results are typically processed by a computer to produce a picture. There is also a way of looking at the tumor directly. The technique is called *endoscopy*. Essentially an endoscope is a long, thin lighted tube acting like a telescope. It is inserted through a body orifice until the far end reaches the suspect area, at which point the physician can see the tumor, usually projected onto a TV screen.

Originally all endoscopic examinations (endoscopies) were done with long, straight, hollow tubes. In recent years, however, flexible endoscopes have been increasingly used, which are made of fiber-optic light pipes allowing light to travel around bends in the tube. Nowadays, flexible endoscopes are used whenever possible and have made endoscopies a distinctly less unpleasant experience.

Endoscopies are generally used whenever the tumor is physically accessible through an appropriate body orifice. As you can imagine, they are not particularly pleasant, but they do allow the physician a direct look at what is happening, which can be a real advantage. Depending on the site, they are either done with a local or general anesthetic.

One of the most common endoscopic procedures is the bronchoscopy, in which a flexible bronchoscope tube is inserted through the mouth or nose to examine some part of the lung. A typical bronchoscopy takes about one hour. Also very common is the colonoscopy, in which a flexible colonoscope is inserted through the rectum to examine the colon.

Sometimes during an endoscopy the physician will also use

a gadget attached to the end of the endoscope to take a sample of the tumor for examination. This technique brings us to the second major type of diagnostic test for cancer, the examination of tissue samples.

Examination of Blood and Tissue Samples

The simplest bodily sample that can be taken is the blood test. Except for blood-related cancers such as leukemia, when a blood test is taken in the context of cancer diagnosis, the aim is not to look for cancer cells themselves, but rather to look for some chemical by-product of the cancer. As molecular studies of cancer become more advanced, it is likely that more and more of these blood tests will be used. The most common and sensitive blood test is for PSA (prostate-specific antigen). All normal prostates in men produce a small amount of PSA, which can be detected in a blood sample, but a cancerous prostate produces much larger quantities, which can easily be detected in a blood sample.

Cytological Studies and Biopsies

Ultimately, the diagnosis of cancer is made by removing and microscopically examining cells taken from the tumor itself. Examination of these cells is usually called a *cytological study*. There are various ways of getting the tumor cells for examination, depending on the location of the tumor. Often the suspicious site is simply scraped to remove some cells. A common example is the so-called Pap smear (named after George Papanicolaou) where the cervix is brushed or scraped to remove cells for examination.

In many cases some possible cancer cells are removed through a *biopsy*. A biopsy is a surgical procedure in which a piece of tissue is removed for examination. Often just a sample of the tumor is removed for examination, in which case the biopsy is called *incisional*. On the other hand, if the tumor is very small, an *excisional* biopsy can be used, where the entire tumor is removed for examination. As well as samples of a suspected tumor, tissue samples in nearby lymph nodes are also often examined.

If the tumor is reasonably accessible, the incisional biopsy is usually performed with a needle. In a needle biopsy, a needle is inserted through the skin into the tumor, and fluid or tissue is drawn out or "aspirated" through the needle. If the potential cancer is less accessible, then a CT scan can be simultaneously taken to allow the needle to be inserted in the exactly right place, a process called CT-guided biopsy. Other options when the cancer is less accessible are an endoscopic biopsy via a bodily orifice, as described above, or a surgical incision.

Once the tumor samples have been taken, it is the job of the pathologist to examine the sample cells. A variety of tests can be performed, but always the aim is to answer four basic questions:

- Are the cells malignant?
- Did the tumor originate in the same organ from which the biopsy was taken, or did it originate somewhere else in the body?
- How abnormal are the cancer cells, and how fast are they growing?
- How advanced is the tumor?

Getting the best answer possible to these questions is extremely important. The most appropriate treatment options are in large part determined by the answers to these questions, so we will look at each of them in more detail.

Are the Cells Malignant?

A growth or tumor can consist of either malignant cells growing out of control, or of benign cells, which are not completely
out of control. As we discussed earlier, malignant cells are
what constitute cancer. By looking at a sample of the cells
under a microscope, a pathologist can normally identify malignant cells, typically by their very disorderly appearance.

Did the Tumor Originate In the
Same Organ from Which the Biopsy Was Taken?

As we discussed earlier, a cancer typically starts growing in one
place in the body, but has the capacity to spread (metastasize)
to other distant parts of the body. By looking at the biopsied
cells under a microscope, the pathologist can usually (though
not always) determine whether the tumor originated in that
location—in which case the tumor is called a *primary tumor*.
On the other hand, if the pathologist determines that the cancer originated in some other part of the body, then it is a *secondary tumor*, and there is probably a primary tumor elsewhere
in the body.

How Fast Is the Tumor Growing?—Its Grade

Malignant tumors can be growing very rapidly, making them
very "aggressive," or they may be growing very slowly, making
them less aggressive. The *grade* of a tumor is a measure of how
aggressive the tumor is. Grade 1 is the least aggressive; grades 3
and 4 are the most aggressive.

The grade, or level of aggression of a tumor, is determined in
one of two ways. The *nuclear grade* describes how fast the cells

are dividing or proliferating. The *histological grade* is a measure of how closely the tumor cells resemble normal cells—grade 1 cells are very similar to normal cells, whereas grade 4 cells look very different from normal cells and tend to grow far more rapidly.

As we will see, the tumor grade is often critical in determining the most appropriate treatment.

How "Advanced" Is the Tumor?—Its Stage

The grade of the tumor describes the state of individual cells in the cancer. The *stage* of the cancer describes the tumor as a whole—how big it is and how much it has spread. More than anything else about the cancer, its stage will determine the possible and the best treatment options.

The advantage of accurate staging of a tumor is that it enables the physician—and you—to make a realistic assessment of the available treatment options. Every tumor and every individual is, of course, unique, but tumors of any given stage share enough common characteristics that it is reasonable to look at groups of people who have had cancer of a particular type and with a particular stage, to get a realistic assessment of the success rates for various treatment options.

Essentially, the stage of a tumor is determined by three factors:

1. The size of the tumor and the degree to which it has spread to nearby healthy tissues.
2. The degree to which the cancer has spread to the nearby lymph nodes. (As we saw in Chapter 1, lymph nodes are part of the body's drainage system for waste products, and cancer cells getting into this lymphatic system can easily be transported to distant parts of the body.)
3. The presence of distant metastases. This means that part of

the primary tumor has broken off and started to grow in other parts of the body. Clearly a cancer growing in several sites is harder to treat than one localized in one place.

These three factors make up the so-called *TNM system* (Tumor size and spread, lymph Node involvement, distant Metastases). The way the system works is that after each letter a number is assigned; the smaller the number, the less advanced is the cancer. So, for example, T1 means a very small primary tumor, while T4 means a large primary tumor or one that has spread to adjacent tissues. N0 means no involvement of lymph nodes, while N3 means major lymph-node involvement. M0 means no distant metastases, while M1 means there are distant metastases.

The actual definition of the stages is different for various types of tumor. So you can't directly compare the severity of, say, a particular stage of breast cancer with a particular stage of lung cancer.

As examples, Table 3.1 shows all the stage definitions for lung cancer. To take a specific case from this table, a T1N0M0 lung cancer would be one in which the primary lung tumor is less than 3 centimeters (1.2 inches) across, has no lymph-node involvement, and has no distant metastases. This would be a less advanced lung cancer case than, say, a T2N1M0 lung cancer, which could be more than 3 centimeters across and have spread to nearby lymph nodes, but has not produced distant metastases.

For the sake of convenience, several of the stages are typically grouped together in "stage groupings." The stage groupings for lung cancer are shown in Table 3.2. For example, a T1N0M0 lung cancer would be a stage I, while a T2N1M0 lung cancer would be a stage II. Again, stage 0 is the least advanced, while stage IV is the most advanced cancer.

TABLE 3.1: TNM System for Classifying Lung Cancers

Tis   Carcinoma *in situ*—very localized

T1   Tumor 3 cm or less in greatest dimension, surrounded by lung or visceral pleura, without bronchoscopic evidence of invasion more proximal than the lobar bronchus

T2   Tumor with any of the following features of size or extent: more than 3 cm in greatest dimension; involves main bronchus, 2 cm or more distal to the carina; invades the visceral pleura; associated with atelectasis or obstructive pneumonitis that extends to the hilar region but does not involve the entire lung

T3   Tumor of any size directly invading any of the following: chest wall, diaphragm, mediastinal pleura, parietal pericardium; or tumor in the main bronchus less than 2 cm distal to the carina but without involvement of the carina; or associated atelectasis or obstructive pneumonitis of the entire lung

T4   Tumor of any size invading any of the following: mediastinum, heart, great vessels, trachea, esophagus, vertebral body, carina; or tumor with a malignant pleural effusion

N0   No regional lymph-node metastasis

N1   Metastasis in ipsilateral peribronchial or ipsilateral hilar lymph nodes, including direct extension

N2   Metastasis in ipsilateral mediastinal or subcarinal lymph node(s)

N3   Metastasis in contralateral mediastinal, contralateral hilar, ipsilateral or contralateral scalene or supraclavicular lymph node(s)

M0   No distant metastasis

M1   Distant metastasis

TABLE 3.2: Grouping of Stages for Lung Cancer

Stage 0	Tis	N0	M0
Stage I	T1	N0	M0
	T2	N0	M0
Stage II	T1	N1	M0
	T2	N1	M0
Stage IIIA	T1	N2	M0
	T2	N2	M0
	T3	N0	M0
	T3	N1	M0
	T3	N2	M0
Stage IIIB	Any T	N3	M0
	T4	Any N	M0
Stage IV	Any T	Any N	M1

Facing Your Diagnosis

Once your diagnosis has been made, and the stage and grade of the cancer have been determined, the next step is to choose the most appropriate treatment. But even before considering treatment options, it is critical to be realistic about your disease. Realistic, here, means facing the central fact that *cancer is a common, serious disease, but it is not an automatic death sentence.*

In the United States today, out of the total population of about 240 million, about 1.2 million people develop cancer every year, and about 8 million people alive today have had cancer at some point in their lives. So it really is a very common disease, and getting more so.

What are the realistic chances of a cure? It depends enormously on the site, the grade, and the stage of the cancer, as we have discussed in this chapter. If all sites, grades, and stages of cancer are averaged together, the chances of surviving five years after the initial diagnosis are a little better than one in two. Depending on the site, low-grade and low-stage cancers generally do better, high grades and stages generally have a worse outlook.

But all these numbers are merely averages. Every person and every cancer is different, and every physician knows of people whose outlook was not considered good, yet who did far better than expected.

The rest of this book is about the options for treating different cancers. The real goal here is to be as informed as possible. Many people have had experiences of talking to physicians (not to mention car mechanics and plumbers!) and coming away from the discussion confused and bewildered. While confusion may not be catastrophic in the case of the car mechanic, it can be in the context of cancer. Understanding what is happening and understanding your realistic options is the best way of ensuring that you and your physicians together will arrive at the most appropriate cancer treatment for you.

And the bottom line here is that getting the most appropriate treatment you can is the best way of stacking the odds in your favor.

Chapter 4

Radiotherapy, Surgery, and Chemotherapy

After all the preliminary tests are done, then comes the time to consider treatment. Radiotherapy, surgery, and chemotherapy have for many years been the mainstay treatments for cancer, and the chances are very high you will end up being treated with one or more of these techniques. In this chapter we will talk about what these three different options are and how they are generally used.

Radiotherapy, surgery, and chemotherapy are by no means the only treatment options available, but they are by far the most common, and the most tested. Surgery is the oldest of the three techniques. What we would now call cancer surgery was being done in Roman times. Radiotherapy has been used since the turn of the twentieth century, while chemotherapy has only been a serious option since the end of World War II.

In recent years there has been an increasing trend toward using more than one of these three basic techniques to treat a cancer. One approach is a combination treatment, where two or even all three techniques are used to attack the tumor. A second approach to multitechnique cancer therapy is what is called adjuvant treatment, where one of the techniques is used to "mop up" a very small number of cells that might have escaped the first, primary treatment.

While this book focuses primarily on radiotherapy, it is also a book about options, and as we shall see, it is absolutely crucial to weigh your possible options if you are to arrive at the most appropriate treatment for you.

Many people reject outright one or more of these treatment options. Certainly, feelings like "under no circumstances would I have chemotherapy" are understandable; every person has a complete right to reject any treatment option. It is, however, important to accept that none of the treatment options can honestly be described as pleasant. It is worth trying to overcome a particular dislike or fear in order to stack the odds as much as possible in your favor.

In large part, the choice between these three techniques (or combination of techniques) depends primarily on the particular type, grade, and stage of the cancer. In this chapter we will briefly describe the basics of the different techniques. The choices between them will be discussed for specific types of cancer in the next chapter.

Radiation Therapy

Radiation therapy, or radiotherapy, is the technique where as much radiation as possible is directed toward a tumor, while exposing healthy normal tissue cells to as little radiation as possible. The most basic rule of radiotherapy is the higher the radiation dose the tumor cells are given, the fewer of them will survive. In order to permanently eradicate a tumor, the goal of radiotherapy is to kill every single tumor cell in the region at which the radiation is directed. Palliative radiotherapy, where the goal is to shrink rather than eradicate the tumor, is discussed later in this chapter.

Essentially, there are two ways of delivering radiation to the tumor. One is called *external* radiotherapy, and the other *internal* radiotherapy or *brachytherapy*.

External Radiotherapy

External radiotherapy (see Fig. 4.1), is so called because the source of the radiation is a machine typically located several feet away, external to the patient. The machine produces a narrow, invisible beam of radiation aimed directly at the tumor. The machine producing the radiation will be moved to several different positions during the course of the treatment, allowing the radiation to reach the tumor from a variety of angles. This cross fire technique reduces the radiation dose that any given healthy tissue receives.

In virtually all cases, radiotherapy treatment is not given all at once, but over an extended period of time. Most often the external beam radiotherapy treatment is divided into thirty or thirty-five daily sessions, or fractions, spread out over six or seven weeks. The reason for this prolonged treatment is to allow time for the body to repair healthy cells damaged by the radiation, which in turn means reduced side effects.

The most common machines used today to produce the radiation for external-beam radiotherapy are either linear accelerators or cobalt-60 machines. Generally, cobalt-60 machines are becoming less and less common, because linear accelerators have the capability to direct more radiation dose into the tumor without increasing the radiation dose to surrounding normal tissues.

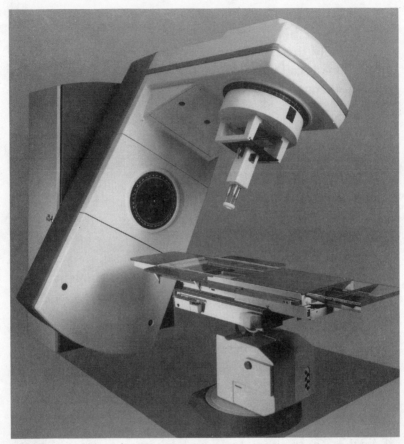

Figure 4.1 A modern radiotherapy machine. The patient lies on the couch, the radiation comes out of the "head" of the machine, and is directed at the tumor. The machine can rotate so as to aim radiation at the tumor from several different directions.

Linear accelerators can produce two different types of radiations—X rays and electrons. Generally, electrons are used for tumors located near the skin, while X or gamma rays are used for more deep-seated tumors, although both are often used in combination.

Internal Radiotherapy—Brachytherapy

Internal radiotherapy uses a series of wires, small "seeds" or pellets made of a material that is constantly emitting gamma rays. These radioactive seeds are physically placed either in the tumor itself or very close to it. The idea here is that because the radioactive seeds are so close to the tumor, the normal tissues receive a much smaller dose of radiation than they would receive during external-beam radiotherapy. Because the distances involved are so much shorter, the treatment is usually called brachytherapy, from the Greek *brachy*, meaning short.

Brachytherapy treatments are also short in time. Because the normal tissues receive a smaller dose than in external-beam radiotherapy, they need less time to recover. Typical treatment times for a complete course of brachytherapy are only a few days, rather than a few weeks.

Of course brachytherapy is only possible when it is practical to place the radioactive seeds in or near the tumor. One way this can be done is if the tumor is close to one of the body cavities, and the radioactive sources can be placed alongside it. This is called *intracavitary brachytherapy*, and the most common examples are for cervical and vaginal cancers, where an applicator containing the radioactive seeds can be placed in the uterus and vagina.

The other way brachytherapy can be done is by implanting the radioactive seeds directly inside the tumor. This is called *interstitial brachytherapy*. It first involves a small surgical procedure in which a series of thin hollow tubes are implanted passing right through the tumor. Inside these metal tubes are flexible plastic tubes, running from the patient across the room to a place called an afterloader, where the radioactive seeds are stored. The radioactive seeds are then shuttled from the afterloader, through the plastic tubes, and stopped at predetermined positions inside the tumor. Typically this sort of treatment takes a few days. One advantage of this afterloader technique is that the radioactive seeds can be temporarily shuttled back out of the patient, allowing friends and family to visit without getting irradiated.

New Types of Radiotherapy

Radiotherapy is a continuously evolving field. New techniques, and variations on old techniques, are constantly being tried out to see if they can produce better results than standard treatments. We will briefly mention a few of the more promising ones now being used to treat cancer, either on an experimental or a more routine basis. Of course, it takes many years before it is possible to judge how good a new treatment option actually is. Most of the new techniques we will describe are sufficiently young and can only be described as promising.

Radiosurgery

This is a radiotherapy technique in which a series of narrow, pencil-sized beams of radiation, under computer control, are aimed, each from a different direction, at a brain tumor. The result is a large amount of radiation can be precisely targeted at the brain tumor, while doing less damage to healthy brain tissues than with conventional radiotherapy. One version of radiosurgery uses the so-called "gamma knife" shown in Figure 4.2. Although it has "surgery" in its name, it does not involve any cutting into the brain, and it can be used to target tumors located deep in the brain and inaccessible to surgery.

Radiosurgery has been used for many years to cure a benign condition in the brain called *arteriovenous malformation*, but it has recently been adapted to treat malignant brain tumors. It is

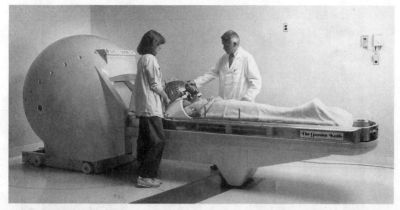

Figure 4.2 The Gamma Knife, one of several types of machines that can be used for radiosurgery, to irradiate brain tumors. The spherical metal shell around the patient's head contains many different radiation sources programmed to direct radiation precisely at the tumor, each from a different direction.

particularly useful for patients who have already received radiotherapy to the brain for a previous cancer. This is because conventional radiotherapy usually can be given only once to the brain, but radiosurgery may be repeated several times if brain tumors recur.

Three-Dimensional Conformal Radiotherapy

This is a technique that involves aiming the radiation, using computer assistance, at the cancer so that the radiation dose conforms to the actual shape of the tumor. This enables both more radiation dose to be given to the cancer, and less unwanted radiation dose to affect the surrounding healthy tissues. An example is shown in Figure 4.3, where the radiation dose is shaped or conformed to the shape of a prostate, thus reducing the amount of radiation received by the nearby bladder and rectum.

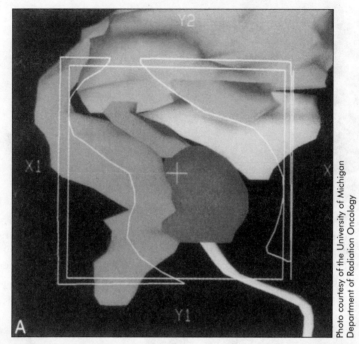

Photo courtesy of the University of Michigan
Department of Radiation Oncology

Figure 4.3 Illustrating the principle of three-dimensional conformal radio-therapy, in this case for prostate cancer therapy. Shown in the picture is the prostate which is the target of the radiotherapy (dark gray area with cross), the rectum (light gray area to the left of the prostate), and the bladder (above the prostate). "Standard" radiotherapy, illustrated by the white square box, as well as the desired irradiation of the prostate, will also irradiate much of the bladder and the rectum. "Conformal" radiotherapy, illustrated by the smaller region outlined in white, conforms the radiation much more closely to just the prostate, so that the bladder and rectum get far less radiation.

Radiolabeled Antibody Therapy

Some of the group of chemicals called antibodies can search out, identify, and attach themselves to cancer cells. When radioactive atoms are attached to these antibodies, radiation can be targeted right at the cancer cells to which the antibodies have attached. This technique, also called *radioimmunotherapy*

(RIT), has achieved some success, mainly as a palliative treatment for advanced cancers.

Radiosensitizers

These are drugs that, when taken into cells, make them more sensitive to killing by radiation. The idea is to attempt to get tumor cells to take up the radiosensitizer, but not normal healthy cells. These drugs are still very much in the experimental stage.

Radioprotectors

These use the opposite approach to radiosensitizers. Here the idea is to use a drug that is taken up by healthy cells in the body, but not the tumor, thus making those cells less sensitive to radiation. In early trials, several chemicals such as misoprostol and prostaglandin have shown some promise for protecting areas like the inside of the mouth during radiotherapy of the head or neck.

Hyperthermia

This is the use of heat: raising the temperature of cells by a few degrees makes them more susceptible to the effects of radiation. Various devices have been made attempting to heat up a tumor (while not heating up surrounding healthy tissues), using ultrasound, microwaves, or radio frequency waves.

Intraoperative radiotherapy

This is a technique of giving a large single dose of radiation to the tumor when it is exposed at the time of surgery. During the operation, the surgeon can temporarily move normal organs to one side so as not to be exposed to the beam directed toward the tumor. The technique can be useful when the tumor is so close to a vital organ that normal radiotherapy would expose the vital organ to too much radiation.

Neutron and Proton Radiation Therapy

While almost all radiotherapy is performed with gamma or X rays, two other types of radiation are being used on an experimental basis: *protons* and *neutrons*. Both these radiations need very expensive multimillion-dollar machines to produce them, so only a few of these machines are being used on a trial basis in the United States. The two types of particles are used for very different reasons: Protons are useful for situations where the radiation dose has to be delivered with exceptional precision. An example is for eye tumors, where any stray radiation would endanger the patient's sight. Neutrons are thought to be useful in situations where a tumor may be very biologically resistant to the effects of X rays. The neutron radiation may be able to overcome this biological resistance, allowing the radiation to kill the tumor cells. Neutrons appear to give better results than X rays for salivary gland tumors, and possibly for prostate cancer and soft-tissue sarcomas, but more studies are needed since neutron treatments are frequently associated with significantly increased damage to healthy normal tissue.

Boron Neutron Capture Therapy (BNCT)

This is a technique being tried out for brain tumors. Boron is a chemical element that reacts strongly with neutron radiation. When this reaction occurs the boron is smashed into small, very damaging fragments. The idea is to put as much boron as possible into a brain tumor, and then aim neutrons at the tumor. When a neutron hits the boron inside a tumor cell, the damaging fragments should then kill that tumor cell. This technique is very much in its trial stages, and only one place in the United States (Brookhaven National Laboratory on Long Island) is using it.

Chemotherapy

Chemotherapy is exactly what the word implies: the use of chemicals for cancer therapy. These chemicals are often referred to as anticancer drugs.

There is one fundamental difference between chemotherapy and either surgery or radiotherapy. While surgery and radiotherapy try to target the primary cancer as much as possible, and aim to affect normal tissues as little as possible, chemotherapy essentially acts on the whole body. Technically this is called a systemic treatment. So while chemotherapy is an option for cancers that have not spread beyond their initial site, it is particularly appropriate when the tumor has spread to other parts of the body.

There is not one "magic" chemotherapy drug that is universally used. In fact more than fifty are in common use. These anticancer drugs often work in different ways from one another, but they all basically address the fact that cancer cells grow and divide very rapidly, so these drugs are aimed at stopping or disrupting the life cycle of the cancer cells in some way.

The two most common types of anticancer drugs are called *antimetabolic drugs* and *alkylating agents*. Antimetabolic drugs basically try to prevent cancer cells from getting the appropriate nutrients they need when they divide, whereas alkylating agents attach to and damage the cells' DNA at all stages of the cells' life cycle. There are a host of other types of anticancer drugs, including hormones, antitumor antibiotics, plant alkyloids, and nitrosureas.

It is now relatively uncommon to use one single anticancer drug. The more common approach is to combine two, three, six, or even more different drugs together, to provide a more potent treatment. This combination is usually described by the first letter of each of the drugs; for example, CMF is a combination of cyclophosphamide, methotrexate, and 5-fluorouracil.

How Are Anticancer Drugs Given?

Essentially there are four ways in which chemotherapy drugs are given: through a vein, by injection into a muscle, by mouth, or topically on the skin. Occasionally the drug may be delivered to one specific organ in the body by means of a catheter tube inserted directly into that organ.

The most common route is through the vein (intravenously, IV). This is sometimes done simply with routine injections into a vein in the arm or hand. Alternately, a thin tube or catheter can be placed into a large vein and left there as long as needed. This catheter is then attached to a device that stores the drug and pumps it into the vein at an appropriate rate. These pumps can be surgically implanted under the skin—which allows for virtually unrestricted activity during treatment—or they can be external. Some external pumps are portable, while others are larger and so rather more restrictive.

How Long Does Chemotherapy Last?

Unlike radiotherapy where most treatments take roughly the same overall time, chemotherapy treatments vary widely in both how long and how often they are given. Chemotherapy is usually given over comparatively long periods of time, usually six months to a year. Some drugs are given daily, some weekly, and some monthly. Often chemotherapy drugs are given in cycles of a few days or weeks, so that the rest period between cycles allows damaged normal cells in the body a chance to recover.

Side Effects

The first question most people ask about chemotherapy relates to side effects. Because anticancer drugs are generally not so directly targeted at the tumor region as with radiotherapy and surgery, significant side effects tend to occur. The drugs are designed to act primarily on rapidly growing cells, and while these include tumor cells, healthy organs in the body also naturally contain rapidly growing cells. These healthy fast-growing normal cells are also damaged by chemotherapy. In particular, the digestive tract, the reproductive system, hair follicles, and blood cells are all generally affected, to a greater or lesser degree, by chemotherapy. On the other hand, it is important to know that not everyone has severe side effects during chemotherapy, and these effects are mostly temporary and start to decrease after the therapy has finished.

Again, as with all cancer treatments, the choice of chemotherapy is a matter of balancing the risks and the benefits. This balance depends upon the particular tumor type in question, as well as its stage and grade, which we discussed in Chapter 3.

Hormone Therapy

Hormone therapy is generally used as an adjuvant (additional) therapy to help stop cancer cells from growing. These hormones are taken either orally or through injections. The basic idea behind hormonal therapy is that some cancer cells, particularly in prostate, breast, and endometrial cancers, need hormones in order to grow. So if the supply of hormones that reach the cancer can somehow be reduced, the tumor should be able to grow less well, and may start to shrink.

For example, adjuvant hormone therapy for breast cancer (usually the drug tamoxifen, see Chapter 6), deprives breast cancer cells of the female hormone estrogen, which some breast cancer cells need to grow. In general, the possible side effects of tamoxifen are similar to those of menopause, such as hot flashes, irregular menstrual periods, vaginal discharge or bleeding, and irritation of the skin around the vagina.

Hormone therapy for prostate cancer (see Chapter 6) basically involves shutting down the body's production of the male hormone testosterone. This can have side effects including hot flashes, loss of libido, occasional loss of potency, breast enlargement, and loss of muscle mass.

Hormone therapy for endometrial cancer generally involves the drug progesterone. This drug usually has few side effects, although some women put on weight. As with tamoxifen, it has a slight tendency to cause blood clots (as do birth control pills as well), so women with a family history of strokes are at some small risk.

Cancer Surgery

Surgery is the oldest form of cancer therapy and perhaps the most intuitive—if there's a lump you don't want, cut it out! Nowadays, cancer surgery is usually done in combination with either radiotherapy or chemotherapy, and sometimes all three are used.

Alhough surgery is the oldest of the three techniques, it is continually developing. A good example is breast cancer surgery. For more than seventy years the radical mastectomy was almost universally used; this involved removal of the entire breast and some surrounding tissues—an exceedingly traumatic operation. Now, breast-conserving surgery is increasingly being used, in combination with radiotherapy, and the success rate currently seems to be every bit as good as for total mastectomy for early-stage breast cancer. Another example is the tremendous improvement in the surgeon's ability to decrease the consequences of the operation, through reconstructive surgery, and also through improved prostheses.

Different Types of Surgery

We talked in Chapter 3 about exploratory surgery to obtain biopsy samples and tumor stage information. Here we briefly discuss so-called "definitive" surgery, where the aim is to remove as much of the tumor as possible.

One important aspect of this kind of surgery is the fact that the surgeon will generally try to remove not only the whole tumor, but also a region or margin of apparently normal tissue surrounding the tumor. Because cancer cells are very invasive, it is possible that a few will have extended slightly beyond what appears to the eye to be the edge of the tumor. If these few cells are not removed, it is possible they could be the starting cells from which the tumor regrows. As well as removing some surrounding tissue, the surgeon will frequently remove some of the lymph nodes (see Chapter 1) in the vicinity of the tumor. This is often done as a preventive measure because of the strong tendency of tumor cells to spread to nearby lymph nodes.

In some situations the tumor is so large, or so close to a vital organ in the body, that it cannot be entirely removed. These tumors are usually called *unresectable*. Surgery, however, often does have a place in treating these tumors. For example, it is used for some brain tumors to remove most of the tumor mass, in a procedure called *debulking*. Alternatively, unresectable tumors are often first treated by radiotherapy or chemotherapy, to shrink them to a point where surgery can remove the entire tumor.

Definitive surgery is a major operation, almost always done under general anesthetic. It typically requires several days' stay in hospital for recovery. As we previously discussed, reconstructive surgery, performed after the primary surgery, is an increasingly important option to produce an end result with which you can be comfortable.

As with chemotherapy and radiotherapy, surgery has its risks and benefits. Again, however, they are very specific to the particular tumor type, as well as its stage and grade, as we shall discuss in the next chapter.

Treating Aggressively—
Curative and Palliative Treatments

The most common (and the most desirable) goal of all types of cancer therapy is a cure, which implies a target of eliminating essentially every single cancer cell. In these *curative* situations, the physician is likely to want to be as aggressive as possible in designing the treatment. In the context of radiotherapy and chemotherapy, this may mean treating with a very high dose—because the higher the dose, the higher the chance of destroying all the cancer cells. In the context of surgery, this may mean removing more apparently normal tissue, to make sure that no cancer cells are left behind.

Inevitably, a more aggressive treatment is going to be less comfortable than a less aggressive treatment. So it is important not to judge the quality of the treatment you are receiving by the degree of discomfort you feel. In the context of radiotherapy and chemotherapy, the most aggressive treatment is one in which the patient is treated "up to normal tissue tolerance"—in other words, the dose is made as high as the patient can possibly tolerate. A less aggressive treatment will be less uncomfortable, but will also likely decrease the chances of completely eradicating the tumor to achieve a complete cure.

There are situations, however, when the goal of cancer therapy cannot be to completely eliminate the cancer. This could be for a variety of reasons, such as the location of the tumor, its size, or the presence of extensive metastases. In this case, the therapy may well be intended to be *palliative* rather than curative. The aim may be, for example, to shrink a tumor so that it does not press on the spinal cord. A palliative treatment, intended to relieve pain or restore some lost function, is typically far less aggressive. The aim is not to treat "up to tolerance," but simply to relieve pain and discomfort when a long-term cure is not likely.

Chapter 5

The Radiotherapy Team

Your radiotherapy treatment will be very much a team effort. During the course of your radiotherapy, you will be meeting and talking to a whole variety of people who are helping with the treatment in some way, and who are talking with each other to get the best possible treatment for you. It is vital to remember the first and most important member of that team is *you*. So it is your right and your responsibility to talk to any and all of the other members of the radiotherapy team.

The Radiation Oncologist

The radiation oncologist is the leader of the team. An oncologist is a physician specializing in treating cancer, so a radiation oncologist is a physician who specializes in treating cancer with radiation. The radiation oncologist holds an M.D. degree or its equivalent, and will also have undergone a three- or four-year training period in the specialty of radiation oncology. Most radiation oncologists then take a special—and difficult—examination through the American Board of Radiology to become certified radiation oncologists.

Being comfortable with your radiation oncologist is the first step to choosing and receiving the best radiotherapy. It is important to note that even the most illustrious hospital does not necessarily have the most famous and competent individual in every medical field, and it is the experience and competence of the individual that matter, not the fame of the institution as a whole. So before signing on as a patient, it is vital to look at the credentials of the radiation oncologist, the leader of the team.

Questions to ask include:

- Is he or she certified in radiation oncology by the American Board of Radiology?
- Is he or she an expert in treating the particular part of the body where your cancer is—breast, lung, prostate, etc.? The techniques for treating different sites in the body are so different that no one can be expert in treating them all. A good question to ask is "How many cancers, of the particular type that I have, have you treated in the last year?"
- You may also want to find out whether he or she keeps up to date with the most recent developments by attending the annual meeting of the American Society for Therapeutic Radiology and Oncology (ASTRO).

As we will see, the radiation oncologist is surrounded by a large support team, but usually the competence of the team reflects the quality of the leader. So be comfortable with your choice of radiation oncologist—a subject we will talk about more in Chapter 8.

The Medical Physicist

The medical physicist is the next member of the radiotherapy team. Radiotherapy equipment is complicated and involves many machines and computers, and the medical physicist is responsible for making sure these are always working optimally. On a day-to-day basis, the medical physicist is responsible for ensuring that the radiation beams are directed to exactly the location the radiation oncologist has specified, and that exactly the right amount of radiation is delivered.

At the center of the medical physicist's profession is quality control. It is the radiotherapist's job to oversee the extensive systems of quality control built into the radiotherapy equipment, including daily checks and measurements of all the key equipment.

A medical physicist has at least a master's degree, and usually a doctorate in physics, followed by several years of apprenticeship in on-the-job clinical training in a radiotherapy department. They are often certified by the American Board of Radiology or the American Board of Medical Physics, a procedure that involves passing a comprehensive series of examinations.

Radiation Therapy Technologists

Radiation therapy technologists (sometimes called radiation therapists) deliver the daily treatments to the patients following the prescription of the radiation oncologist, and under his/her supervision. Since they see the patient on a daily basis, they are the first to spot a problem, and it is their responsibility to maintain daily records and alert the physicist or engineer if the treatment machines are not working properly. This is a "people's job" since the technologist can do a great deal to help and reassure the cancer patient every day.

Radiation therapy technologists complete a two- or four-year educational program following high school, which in some cases includes a bachelor's degree. They must then pass a special examination and can be accredited by the American Registry of Radiologic Technologists. In addition, many states require that radiation therapy technologists be licensed. In the United States, radiation therapy technologists have their own national society (the American Society of Radiation Technologists, ASRT), which meets in parallel with the American Society of Radiation Oncologists, in order to benefit from the refresher courses and educational opportunities.

Dosimetrists

Dosimetrists work under the supervision of the radiation oncologist and the medical physicist, and their chief duty is treatment planning. This means that for each individual patient, they perform detailed and complicated calculations to determine how best to aim and arrange the beams of radiation to destroy the tumor while minimizing damage to surrounding healthy tissues. These calculations, which are performed with a computer, are always double- and triple-checked to be certain they are correct. Some dosimetrists start as technologists, others with a bachelor's degree in physics, while others take a two-year dosimetry program following high school: Whatever their background, on-the-job training and experience are then required. Dosimetrists can be certified through the Medical Dosimetrist Certification Board.

Radiation Therapy Nurses

Radiation therapy nurses are often your best point of contact with the radiotherapy team on a day-to-day basis. One of their main jobs is to help educate patients and their families about what is likely to happen during the course of radiation treatment. They can discuss possible side effects and the many other worries and concerns that go along with cancer treatment. In short, they provide emotional support to cancer patients and their families. In addition, they regularly weigh you, take your blood pressure, and generally help maintain your health during the course of your radiotherapy. Radiation therapy nurses have completed a registered nursing program, successfully passed the required written examinations, and are licensed to practice as nursing professionals.

Dietitians

Dietitians work with you to ensure you eat well and appropriately during the radiotherapy. They monitor your weight on a regular basis, and can suggest recipes and/or vitamin supplements to maintain your nutritional status. As we shall see, eating well is a very important part of coping with a course of radiotherapy. Dietitians usually have a bachelor's degree, followed by a one-year internship. They are often certified by the American Dietetic Association.

Social Workers

Social workers can be an enormously important part of the team. It almost goes without saying that the emotional strain of coping with cancer, and coping with cancer treatment, are enormous. Social workers are there to provide support for patients and their families who, for any number of reasons, may be depressed or anxious. As well as emotional issues, they can advise on home health care, help to arrange transportation, or help arrange accommodation during treatment away from home. Licensed social workers must pass an examination following a bachelor's or master's degree and two years of practical experience.

Support Groups

Support groups are designed to help their members explore and share their feelings about the problems they are facing and many hospitals organize them. Some groups meet only for the length of the hospital stay, while others are long-term for discussing the problems of returning to everyday life. Some of these groups are just for patients, while others include family members and friends. Support groups offer an opportunity to share feelings, fears, and anxieties with other people who are in similar situations. Often they provide a place where people can express feelings they feel would be a burden to family and friends. These groups also provide an opportunity to exchange tips and hints garnered through the experience of "being there," as well as give support and information to help patients, families, and friends gain some control over their lives. As well as being organized through hospitals, there are many local and national support groups; more recently, support groups have been formed through electronic mail. More information on locating these groups is given in Appendix D.

Chapter 6

The Most Common Cancers: What Are Your Options?

In this chapter, we talk in detail about treatment options for the most common cancers. Rather than list all the possibilities, we will talk only about the more realistic and common options. In many cases, the choice is pretty clear—one treatment option is much better than any others. Often, however, the choice is less clear, and depends on many factors, not least of which is your own personal preference.

After you read the section for your particular cancer, you should have enough information to join with your physicians in arriving at the treatment option that is right for you.

This chapter by no means covers all of the more than one hundred different cancers. The ones we have chosen are here, first, because they are the most common and, second, because they are most commonly treated with radiation therapy.

Breast Cancer

Breast cancer is the most common of all cancers in women in Western countries, representing about one-third of all women's cancers. In 1995, more than 180,000 American women were diagnosed with breast cancer, and more than 45,000 died from this disease. In the United States about one woman in eight will develop breast cancer at some point in her life. Although cure rates are improving, breast cancer is still the leading cause of cancer death in women under fifty, and the second leading cause of cancer death in women of all ages, after lung cancer. The disease also occurs, but very rarely, in men, accounting for less than 1 percent of all breast cancer cases.

The female breast is an extraordinarily complex organ. Basically (Fig. 6.1), it is made up of the glands that manufacture milk (called *lobules*), tiny tubes for the milk to reach the nipple (called *ducts*), as well as soft connective tissue and fat. Underneath the breast are chest muscles, which cover the ribs.

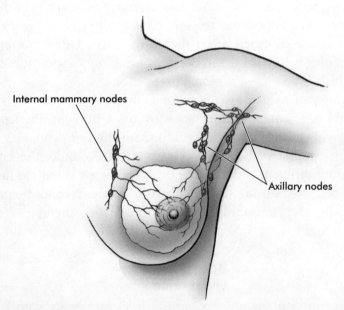

Figure 6.1 The female breast and the different lymph nodes that can be involved in breast cancer.

Breast cancer, at least when it is detected at a relatively early stage, is a disease for which there are realistic alternative therapies from which to choose. The determining factors will be your own personal preferences, the type of cancer, its stage, and its grade. As we discussed in Chapter 3, the stage of the cancer covers a variety of factors including the tumor size, whether it has spread to nearby lymph nodes, and whether there are metastases in other parts of the body.

Types of Breast Cancer

The first distinction, in terms of types of breast cancer, is between invasive and noninvasive cancers. In general, most cancers, by their nature, are invasive, meaning that they tend to grow into surrounding healthy tissue. Sometimes, however, early in a cancer's development, it is apparently not growing into the surrounding tissues, in which case it is called *in situ*, meaning staying at one site. About one in seven of all breast cancers fall into this category.

A noninvasive breast cancer can be ductal carcinoma *in situ* (DCIS) or lobular cancer *in situ* (LCIS), depending upon whether it originated in the breast ducts (through which breast milk travels) or the lobules (the milk-producing glands). If not treated, DCIS is likely to develop into an invasive tumor, whereas LCIS may not. In fact, only about one in four untreated LCIS cases will develop into an invasive tumor, and so LCIS is often not classified as a cancer at all.

The remaining six out of seven breast cancers are invasive, and therefore more immediately threatening. Just as with *in situ* cancers, they are usually divided between ductal and lobular. By far the most common breast cancer is *invasive ductal cancer*, accounting for approximately 70 percent of all breast cancers.

These cancers generally show up as a lump—a feeling a bit like a pebble or stone when you squeeze or palpate the breast.

The next most common infiltrating cancer is *infiltrating lobular cancer*, which accounts for about 5 to 10 percent of all breast cancers. Unlike the lumpy characteristics of infiltrating ductal carcinomas, these lobular carcinomas tend to show up as a general thickening of the breast, and often in several different places—including the opposite breast. In terms of treatment, infiltrating ductal and lobular carcinomas have about the same success rate.

Although there are several other types of breast cancer, they are all rare. Combinations of cancer types are quite common, however, including a mixture of *in situ* and invasive cancers.

As we saw in Chapter 3, physicians use a standard "TNM" system to describe the seriousness or stage of a particular cancer. T is for tumor size, N is for cancer in nearby lymph nodes, and M is for the presence of metastases. Many of the preliminary tests done before the treatment options are decided are aimed toward defining the stage of the cancer, because it is such an important factor to consider when deciding on the best treatment option.

Simply as a convenience, some of the T, N, and M combinations are usually grouped together, as shown in Table 6.1, into six stages, described (from least to most serious) as 0, I, II, IIIA, IIIB, and IV. Here stage 0 corresponds to *in situ* cancer. Happily, the lower stages are the most common, and this trend is increasing with mammography providing earlier diagnosis of breast cancer. Currently, more than half of all breast cancers are in stage 0 or I. Generally the treatment options and outlook are fairly similar within each one of these six groups.

All three TNM factors are very important. Small tumors generally have a better outlook than larger tumors, and evidence

TABLE 6.1. Simplified Stages of Breast Cancer

	Tumor Size?	Cancer In Lymph Nodes?	Metastases In Distant Parts of the Body?
Stage 0	*In situ* cancer—very localized	No	No
Stage I	Tumor no bigger than ¾" (2 cm) across	No	No
Stage II	Tumor is more than 1" across, but has not reached chest wall or skin	Tumor may have spread to reach axillary (underarm) lymph nodes	No
Stage IIIA	Tumor can be any size but has not reached the chest wall or skin	Tumor has spread to the axillary (underarm) lymph nodes, and may have caused these to grow and attach to each other and to other nearby tissues	No
Stage IIIB	Tumor can be any size and may have reached the chest wall or skin	Tumor may have reached lymph nodes near the breastbone as well as underarm	No
Stage IV	Tumor can be any size	Tumor probably has spread to lymph nodes	Yes

of cancer in lymph nodes is often important in deciding on the best treatment. The closest lymph nodes to the breast are the "axillary" lymph nodes, located in the armpit. Typically, several axillary lymph nodes are removed and examined during cancer surgery. As we shall discuss later in this section, the outcome of the examination of these lymph nodes is important in determining whether adjuvant (extra) therapy is an appropriate option. As we saw earlier, it is not the presence of cancer cells in the lymph nodes themselves that is the cause for concern, but rather the fact that, once there, the cancer cells have the potential to spread to other parts of the body through the lymphatic system.

Tumor Grade

As discussed in Chapter 3, your biopsy will enable the pathologist to grade the tumor cells as to how aggressively they will grow. Grades range from 1, where the cells are not that different from normal healthy cells, to grade 3, where the cells are highly abnormal and growing very aggressively.

Estrogen Receptor and Progesterone Receptor Status

Another factor that often plays a large role in the outcome of the treatment is whether the breast cancer cells are estrogen-receptor positive, progesterone-receptor positive, or both. If either of these tests is positive, it means the cancer cells are using the hormone estrogen in order to grow. If this is the case, then hormone therapy, which blocks the tumor cells' use of estrogen, becomes a reasonable option.

Treatment Options

Before discussing the most appropriate treatment choices for your particular breast cancer, let us first review the main treatment options available. Basically, three types of treatment (or combinations of these three types) are commonly used:

- Surgery (removing the cancer in an operation)
- Radiation therapy (using radiation to kill cancer cells)
- Chemotherapy (using drugs to kill cancer cells), and/or hormone therapy (using hormones to stop tumor cells from growing)

There are other options, such as biological therapy (using your body's immune system to fight cancer) and bone marrow transplantation, both of which are being tested in clinical trials.

Surgery for Breast Cancer

For all but very advanced cancers, surgery is almost certain to be part of the final treatment decision. There are two basic kinds of surgical procedures for removing the cancer: breast-conserving surgery done in combination with radiotherapy, and non-breast-conserving surgery. We will discuss the pros and cons of the two approaches later in this section. For now, we describe what the two surgical options actually are.

The Breast-Conserving Option: Lumpectomy and Radiotherapy

In this option, the tumor lump is surgically removed, as well as some surrounding breast tissue. The operation is called a *lumpectomy*, because the prime goal is to remove the tumor lump. It is also called a partial or segmental mastectomy, depending upon how much normal breast tissue is removed. Generally, in these operations, some lymph nodes are removed from under the armpit (this is called an axillary dissection), and a course of radiotherapy almost always follows the surgery. The lumpectomy is becoming increasingly common: in 1987 it was used in about one-third of all breast cancer surgeries. By 1992, it was used in almost half of all breast cancer surgeries.

The Non-Breast-Conserving Option: Mastectomy

The most common operation of this type is called the *modified radical mastectomy*. This involves removal of the entire breast, the breast lining above the chest muscles, and sometimes, one of the two chest muscles. As with lumpectomy, some lymph nodes under the armpit are also removed. This operation is still the most common treatment for breast cancer, and is now often done in tandem with breast reconstructive surgery. There are other non-breast-conserving operations, such as the total mastectomy, where less chest muscle and lining are removed, and the radical, or Halsted, mastectomy, where the breast and all the chest muscles are removed; although the radical mastectomy is now quite rare. Except for unusual situations or very advanced cancers, radiotherapy is generally not used after non-breast-conserving surgery. Non-breast-conserving surgery generally requires a stay in hospital of several days.

Radiotherapy for Breast Cancer

The most common role of radiotherapy in treating breast cancer is as an integral part of the breast-conserving surgery option. Breast-conserving surgery without radiotherapy is almost never done because of the risk that some cancer cells might not have been removed during the lumpectomy. Probably more than one-quarter of all lumpectomies leave some cancer cells behind. The radiotherapy is designed kill those few tumor cells remaining.

Radiotherapy treatment typically starts a few weeks after surgery, and involves daily treatments (excluding weekends) for five or six weeks. Each treatment session lasts only a few minutes. Generally, the radiotherapy course consists of two parts. In the first part, the entire breast is treated with radiation, but toward the end of the radiotherapy course, a "boost" is given, where the radiation is aimed only at the region from which the tumor was removed.

The second major use of radiotherapy in breast cancer is as adjuvant (additional) therapy after a modified radical mastectomy (non-breast-conserving surgery). This is by no means always necessary, but is used in those situations where it seems likely some of the cancer has spread beyond the breast to the chest wall or the skin. It is also usually used if a considerable number of tumor cells were found in the lymph nodes. Adjuvant radiotherapy would be a reasonable option, for example, if the primary cancer was very large, or when the edge of the tissue that had been removed showed signs of cancer cells, or when several lymph nodes showed signs of cancer.

Chemotherapy and Hormone Therapy for Breast Cancer

Generally, chemotherapy and hormonal therapy are adjuvant (additional) treatments for breast cancer. They are added on either to surgery, or to surgery and radiotherapy. There are some very aggressive breast cancers for which chemotherapy is used as the primary treatment, but this is quite unusual.

Because chemotherapy and hormone therapy act over the whole body (technically, called systemic action), they are reasonable options to add to radiotherapy when there is a significant chance that the cancer has spread beyond the breast. Thus, very early stage cancer such as stage 0 (*in situ* cancer) or very small stage 1 cancers are often not treated with additional chemotherapy or hormonal therapy. Larger or more advanced tumors, on the other hand, often are treated with additional hormone therapy, chemotherapy, or both. Additional chemotherapy is also increasingly being used for premenopausal women at particular risk (as indicated, for example, by a high tumor grade) for developing metastases.

As we saw in Chapter 4, chemotherapy treatments usually consist of combinations of several drugs, the most common combination being CMF (cyclophosphamide, methotrexate, and 5-fluorouracil). Typically, the chemotherapy drugs are given for about six months in monthly cycles, each cycle consisting of two weeks taking the drugs and a two-week break without the drugs.

If chemotherapy is given as an adjuvant to the lumpectomy/radiotherapy option, the question arises in what order the radiotherapy and chemotherapy should be given. The straight answer is that we really don't know. Various options have been tried, such as radiotherapy followed by chemotherapy, or chemotherapy followed by radiotherapy, or starting the two together, or having a chemotherapy-radiotherapy-chemotherapy "sandwich." There are no very convincing data to suggest one way is better than another. Probably the most desirable option is to start the chemotherapy and the radiotherapy together, although with some chemotherapy cocktails this combination can be quite hard to tolerate. The next most desirable option is probably having chemotherapy followed by radiotherapy but, again, the definitive answer really is not known.

The most common hormone drug for breast cancer patients

is tamoxifen, which is simply taken as a daily pill. Tamoxifen prevents cancer cells from using the body's natural estrogen, which the cells often need in order to grow. It is most commonly used for women who have gone through menopause, and is rarely used for women under fifty. When hormone therapy is used, it needs to be taken over a long period of time—at least two or three years, and often for five years.

Breast-Sparing Surgery and Radiation vs. Non-Breast-Sparing Surgery

This is the major choice facing most women who have breast cancer in its earlier stages. Since most women with breast cancer are diagnosed when it is in these early stages, most women with breast cancer will be faced with this decision.

The breast-sparing surgery option is a comparatively new one, and it was only in 1990 that the National Institutes of Health concluded that

> . . . breast conservation treatment is an appropriate method of primary therapy for the majority of women with stage I and II breast cancer and is preferable because it provides survival equivalent to total mastectomy and axillary dissection while preserving the breast.

How did they come to this conclusion? It came on the basis of six large studies, worldwide, in which women with stage I or II breast cancer agreed to be given either breast-sparing surgery and radiotherapy, or modified radical mastectomy (surgical removal of the breast). In total, about 4,000 women participated in the trials—about 1,500 in the United States, 700 in Italy, 600 in Denmark, 200 in France, and 900 in a European study. Half of the women received breast-sparing surgery and radiotherapy, and the other half had a modified radical mastectomy.

The results of these studies are very clear: There is essentially no difference in outcome between the two options for women with stage I or II breast cancer. This is illustrated in Figure 6.2, where the survival rate is given for the women in each of the trials, both for women who had breast-sparing surgery and radiotherapy, and for women who had a mastectomy.

Of course, statistics are only one of the factors affecting your decision. As we will talk about further, women who are faced with this decision usually experience many different emotions. Frequently, being told that lumpectomy and radiation is "as

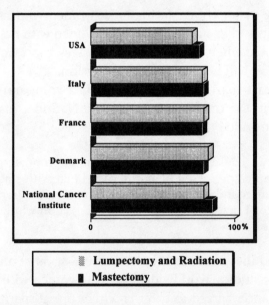

Figure 6.2 The results of different large clinical trials around the world comparing the outcome of the breast-sparing option (lumpectomy and radiation) with the non breast-sparing option (mastectomy). The results, for early-stage breast cancer, show quite clearly that there is no difference in the outcome of the two treatments in terms of long term survival.

good" simply does not satisfy the very real emotional and psychological need to have the "cause" of the disease—the breast—removed. Of course, pulling in the other direction are the very real cosmetic and emotional advantages of conserving the breast. Ultimately it must come down to your decision, but the key fact to keep in mind is that both options control the disease equally well.

DCIS (ductal cancer *in situ*—stage 0 cancer) is a much rarer disease, and so has not been subject to such large-scale studies. One thing is clear, as with stage I and II breast cancers, a breast-sparing operation *without* radiotherapy is not a good option. It does appear likely that, for most women with DCIS, the breast-sparing option with radiotherapy is as good an option as a mastectomy, but there are occasions when the DCIS is too large to be adequately removed, in which case a mastectomy is a more reasonable option.

Choosing the Right Treatment Option for Your Breast Cancer

Now is the time to weigh the choices that are going to be presented to you. We will go through the various stages of breast cancer to see what are the realistic options:

Stage 0 In Situ *Cancer*

For DCIS (ductal carcinoma *in situ*), the outlook is excellent, with more than 95 percent of all women living more than five years. As we saw, the two main options are breast-conserving surgery followed by radiation, or a total mastectomy. In general, the breast-conserving option is likely to be appropriate, although on rare occasions when the disease is too extensive to be adequately removed, total mastectomy is a very safe alternative.

For LCIS (lobular carcinoma *in situ*), there has been a shift in the preferred treatment option since the 1960s. At that time the most common option was total mastectomy, usually of both breasts. Now the most common option is to have no treatment, but simply to wait and watch, with mammographic examinations perhaps twice each year. This watch-and-wait approach is perfectly appropriate except for those people who would find it too stressful to know there is about a one in four chance that an invasive cancer will be found one day. For those women, the mastectomy option may be better for their peace of mind. One issue here is that the most appropriate mastectomy procedure for women with LCIS is of *both* breasts, because the chances of developing invasive cancer are as high in the breast without LCIS as in the breast with it.

Stage I Breast Cancer

The two main options are lumpectomy followed by radiation (the breast-conserving option), and a modified radical mastectomy (the non-breast-conserving option). The treatment is often supplemented by chemotherapy or hormone therapy.

As we have seen, there is very strong evidence that for stage I cancers the success rate is essentially the same for lumpectomy followed by radiation, as for a modified radical mastectomy. In general then, the choice must be yours. As one would expect, studies have shown that women who undergo breast-conserving treatment have more positive feelings about their bodies and undergo fewer changes in their feelings of sexual desirability, compared with women who have a mastectomy.

In some unusual situations, breast-conserving surgery and radiotherapy is not a good option. One is during the first six months of pregnancy, because the radiation will almost certainly damage the growing fetus. During late pregnancy, however, lumpectomy is an option, because the radiotherapy can be delayed until after the baby is born. Another situation when lumpectomy is often not a good option is when there are several lumps in different parts of the breast. The combination of a small breast and a large tumor also tends to make lumpectomy a less attractive option, as removal of the lump might lead to an unacceptable cosmetic outcome, in which case a mastectomy followed by breast reconstruction would be a better option.

Two other situations can make radiotherapy—and thus the breast-conserving option—difficult. One is if the breast is very large and pendulous; this makes radiotherapy with conventional machines difficult to do, although some radiotherapy centers have developed specialized techniques for properly irradiating a very large breast. Finally, if for some reason the breast has undergone radiotherapy before, it is often not possible to expose it to radiotherapy a second time.

Stage II Breast Cancer

The options for stage II breast cancer are essentially the same as those for stage I, and the same considerations apply to the choice between breast-conserving surgery plus radiotherapy, and radical mastectomy.

Adjuvant chemotherapy or hormone therapy is often given for stage II cancers, in addition to the primary treatment. Often, both these additional treatments are given, although for elderly women, hormone therapy without chemotherapy is the recommended choice.

Stage IIIA Breast Cancer

The standard treatment for stage IIIA breast cancer is a modified radical mastectomy. If the cancer has spread to the chest muscles, then a full radical mastectomy is a better option. For stage IIIA cancers, breast-conserving surgery is not a practical option, because of the larger size of the tumor.

After surgery for stage IIIA breast cancer, adjuvant treatment is essential, and the most promising results have been obtained with a combination of surgery, radiotherapy, and chemotherapy. The role of hormone therapy in addition to radiotherapy and chemotherapy is not clear at this point, although it is unlikely to be harmful.

Occasionally, either radiotherapy or chemotherapy is given before surgery, but usually only to shrink the tumor somewhat in those situations where the tumor is so large as to border on being inoperable.

Stage IIIB Breast Cancer

Stage IIIB cancers are usually either inoperable or on the borderline of being inoperable. After a biopsy, the most common treatment is a combination of radiotherapy and chemotherapy. If the tumor shrinks during the treatment, then a mastectomy may be a reasonable possibility.

Many new approaches are being tried for very advanced breast cancers, such as bone marrow transplantation in combination with aggressive chemotherapy, although these approaches are still very much in the trial stage.

Stage IV Breast Cancer

Because of the need to control distant metastases, chemotherapy and hormonal therapy are the primary treatments for stage IV breast cancer, which, fortunately, is extremely rare. If practical, the primary tumor can be treated with surgery or radiation. Again, many new approaches are being tried for very advanced breast cancers, such as bone marrow transplantation in combination with aggressive chemotherapy, although these approaches are still very much in the trial stage. Because five-year survival levels for stage IV breast cancer are not encouraging—around 10 percent—seeking out a trial of a new therapy is not an unreasonable option.

Prostate Cancer

Prostate cancer is an exceedingly common disease. In 1994, prostate cancer overtook lung cancer as the most frequently diagnosed cancer (other than skin cancer) among American men, with an estimated 200,000 new cases. In 1995, there were an estimated 244,000 new cases. About 40,000 men die from prostate cancer every year in the United States.

Currently, a fifty-year-old American man has about a 40 percent chance of developing prostate cancer, a 10 percent chance of actually being diagnosed with prostate cancer, and about a 2 percent chance of dying of the disease. More and more prostate cancers are being diagnosed. One estimate suggests that by the year 2000, the number of prostate cancers diagnosed each year in the United States will be almost double the number in 1990.

The prostate is a male sex gland, part of the reproductive system. Its job is in the making of seminal fluid. The prostate is about the size of a walnut and located below the bladder, close to the front wall of the rectum (see Fig. 6.3). The prostate surrounds the upper portion of the urethra, which is the tube that carries urine from the bladder.

Prostate cancer is usually diagnosed in one of two ways. One way is if symptoms appear—often problems with urination, particularly a weak or interrupted flow of urine, urinating too often, pain while urinating, or blood in the urine. The first

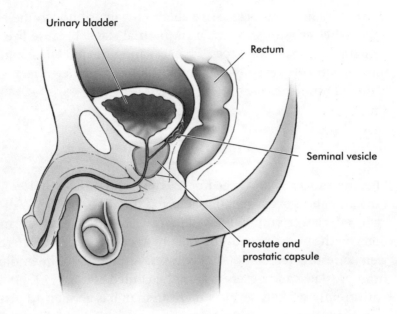

Urinary bladder

Rectum

Seminal vesicle

Prostate and
prostatic capsule

Figure 6.3. The prostate and surrounding organs

test your physician will give you will probably be a rectal exam, in which the doctor inserts a gloved finger into the rectum to feel for lumps in the prostate. If a lump is found, a biopsy would be the next step.

The other way to diagnose prostate cancer is through a routine screening test. Nowadays it is recommended that all men over the age of forty or fifty have their prostate checked during an annual routine checkup. These checkups are typically done both with a rectal exam, as we have seen, and with a comparatively new tool called the PSA test.

PSA stands for prostate-specific antigen. Normal prostate cells make this chemical, and it ends up in the bloodstream, where it can be measured as part of a routine blood test. Cancerous prostate cells, however, make PSA much more rapidly than normal, so the PSA level in the blood is much higher. Typical PSA levels in the blood of men who do not have prostate cancer range from about 2.5 units (technically, 2.5 nanograms per milliliter of blood) for a man in his forties to about 6.5 units for a man in his seventies. A measurement much higher than this average is a very strong indication there may be prostate cancer. It is important to realize, however, that a high PSA reading does not automatically mean cancer. Benign prostate growths, which can also cause urinary problems, also result in high PSA readings. The real danger signal is a PSA reading that rises significantly from one test to the next.

It is probable that the advent of the PSA test, which became common only in the late 1980s, is mostly responsible for the tremendous increase in the number of prostate cancers being diagnosed. This means that prostate cancers are being caught earlier and earlier.

Stages and Grades of Prostate Cancer

Just as with all other cancers, prostate cancers are grouped together by their stage (how advanced they are), and their grade (how aggressive the tumor cells are). While the standard TNM system (tumor size, nodal involvement, metastases) is increasingly used for prostate cancer stages, a simpler "ABCD" is still frequently used; the different stages are categorized in Table 6.2.

In 1990, about 30 percent of diagnosed prostate cancers were of stage A, 38 percent were stage B, 12 percent were stage C, and 20 percent were stage D.

The grade of the prostate cancer, a measure of how aggressively the cancer cells are growing, is usually scored on a scale of 2 to 10, called the Gleason scale. The least aggressive are Gleason scores of 2 to 4, where the cells are not much different

Table 6.2: Simplified Stages of Prostate Cancer

Old System	TNM System	
Stage A1	T1a (N0M0)	Tumor not large enough to be felt during a rectal exam. Three or fewer regions of microscopic tumor found.
Stage A2	T1b and T1c (N0M0)	Tumor not large enough to be felt. More than three regions of microscopic tumor found.
Stage B	T2 (N0M0)	Tumor large enough to be felt, but has not spread beyond the prostate.
Stage C	T3 (N0M0)	Tumor has spread beyond the prostate.
Stage D	N1, N2, N3, or M1	Tumor has reached lymph nodes, or metastasized to distant parts of the body.

from normal cells. Scores of 5 to 7 are considered moderately aggressive, and scores of 8 to 10 are considered very aggressive.

Treatment Options for Prostate Cancer

There are essentially four main options for the treatment of prostate cancer:

- doing nothing but watching the cancer closely
- radiotherapy
- surgical removal of the prostate
- hormone therapy

As with all cancers, the choices depend very much upon the stage and grade of the cancer, as well as your age and overall health. In the rest of this section we will outline various treatments and discuss realistic options for different situations.

The choice of treatment for prostate cancer changed dramatically in the late 1980s and early 1990s, as illustrated in Figure 6.4. The most striking change is the dramatic increase in the proportion of men with prostate cancer opting for surgery to remove the prostate. In 1985 surgical removal of the prostate (prostatectomy) was used in less than 10 percent of all prostate cancer treatments, but by 1992 it was used in more than 30 percent of all treatments.

The increase in the use of surgery to remove the prostate is a source of much controversy. After we describe the main therapy options, we will discuss the issues involved in the increased use of the prostatectomy. Finally, we will discuss the most realistic options, stage by stage.

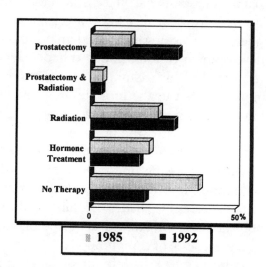

Figure 6.4 Treatment patterns for prostate cancer in 1985 and in 1992. The main difference is that far more men are opting for the prostatectomy operation while less men are choosing the "wait-and-watch" option. Whether this trend makes good sense is yet unclear.

Radiotherapy for Prostate Cancer

Radiotherapy was first used to treat prostate cancer as long ago as 1910. It is not the easiest of cancers to treat with radiotherapy because of the fact (see Fig. 6.3) that the bladder and rectum are extremely close to the prostate. So the mark of a good radiotherapy treatment is to give as much radiation dose as possible to the cancer, while giving as little radiation dose as possible to the bladder and rectum.

As discussed in Chapter 4, radiotherapy can be given in two ways, externally or internally. Internal radiotherapy (brachytherapy), involving the insertion of radioactive seeds or ribbons directly into the tumor, was very popular a few years ago for treating prostate cancer. Its popularity is increasing once again because it reduces the radiation dose to the bladder and rectum, which in turn should lead to lessened side effects.

In external beam radiotherapy (see Chapter 4), the source of radiation is a machine (usually a linear accelerator) located outside the patient. The big advance in external radiotherapy has been the development of a technique called *three-dimensional conformal radiotherapy*. This technique, which is most appropriate for tumors confined to the prostate itself, involves aiming the radiation (assisted by computer) at the prostate so that the radiation dose conforms to the actual shape of the prostate being treated. This enables more radiation dose to be given to the cancer, while decreasing unwanted radiation dose to the bladder and rectum. In principle, at least, more radiation dose to the prostate increases the chance of killing all the cancer cells in the tumor—and less radiation dose to the bladder and rectum decreases the chance of complications.

A typical radiotherapy schedule for prostate cancer would involve daily treatments (excluding weekends) for about six to eight weeks. In general, the radiotherapy is scheduled as soon as practical after that treatment option has been chosen.

We discuss side effects more in Chapter 7, but generally they are tolerable after prostate radiotherapy and can be well treated with medication. The most common side effects of radiotherapy are diarrhea, occuring in roughly 1 in 10 patients, and rectal inflammation (proctitis), occuring in roughly 1 in 20 patients. These side effects tend to start a few weeks after treatment begins and subside a few weeks after treatment finishes. In about 1 in 50 patients, however, the side effects occur much later and are sufficiently severe that surgery is needed to repair damage to the bladder or rectum. The numbers quoted here are for external radiotherapy done without using the three-dimensional conformal technique (this new approach reduces complication levels somewhat). The complication rates after internal radiotherapy (brachytherapy) are considerably lower than those from external radiotherapy.

Sexual potency can be affected by radiotherapy for prostate cancer. Roughly half of all men treated with external-beam radiotherapy for prostate cancer lose their sexual potency. Again, three-dimensional conformal radiotherapy should reduce these numbers, but the technique is sufficiently new that the degree of benefit has not yet been proven. As with other side effects, loss of potency is considerably less common after internal radiotherapy (brachytherapy).

After radiotherapy, loss of potency is not sudden, but may occur slowly over several years. This is in contrast to surgery, where, if potency is lost, which is commonly the case, it happens immediately. Clearly, loss of potency is a very important consideration, and we will come back to it when we compare radiotherapy with surgery—the other possible option for treatment of prostate cancer.

Surgery for Prostate Cancer

Radical prostatectomy involves the complete surgical removal of the prostate and some surrounding tissue. The basic idea behind this surgery is that if the cancer is completely confined within the prostate gland, removal of the prostate should result in a complete cure. The operation was pioneered in Baltimore in the 1900s, but did not become common until the 1980s.

The operation may be done by cutting into the region between the scrotum and the anus (the perineum); this is called a perineal prostatectomy. More commonly, an incision is made into the lower abdomen, and the operation is then called a retropubic prostatectomy.

The first step in a radical prostatectomy operation is an examination of the pelvic lymph nodes. If there are cancer cells in the lymph nodes, the operation will usually be terminated and the prostate will not be removed, because the cancer is too far spread for the surgery to be successful.

As we mentioned, the radical prostatectomy became much more common in the 1980s. This is largely because of the development of the so-called "nerve-sparing" prostatectomy by Patrick Walsh at Johns Hopkins Hospital in Baltimore. Attached to the prostate are two neurovascular bundles controlling sexual potency—man's ability to have an erection. Before the nerve-sparing operation, these bundles were severed during a prostatectomy, almost always leading to impotency.

The nerve-sparing prostatectomy is an extremely delicate procedure in which either or both of the neurovascular bundles are separated from the prostate, after which the prostate is removed. The procedure is difficult and controversial. Some of the time, attempts to spare the nerves will also lead to sparing the cancer—in other words, not all of the tumor gets removed. How often this occurs will depend to a considerable extent on the skill of the surgeon; estimates vary from one time in two, up to one time in twenty.

The two main side effects associated with surgery are incontinence (leaking of urine) and impotence. In addition, there are risks associated with undergoing general anesthesia and a major surgical procedure. The biggest study of complications in men across the United States was a national survey of Medicare patients who underwent radical prostatectomy between 1988 and 1990. In that survey, about one-third of men reported the need for pads or clamps for urinary wetness, and two-thirds reported a current problem with wetness. Six out of ten men reported having no erections since surgery, and nine out of ten had no erections sufficient for intercourse during the month prior to the survey. In other words, surgery generally produces similar or rather higher impotency rates compared with radiotherapy, and considerably higher rates of incontinence.

Hormone Suppression Therapy for Prostate Cancer

For advanced prostate cancer, hormone suppression therapy is the most common therapy. The idea behind hormone therapy is the fact that some (although not all) prostate cancer cells need, for their growth, male sex hormone chemicals called *androgens*. Most of the body's supply of androgens comes via testosterone, which is made in the testicles. So if the supply of androgens can be reduced or removed, most of the prostate cancer cells should die, or stop growing.

The main techniques currently used to reduce the supply of androgens to the prostate are LHRH agonist drugs and an anti-androgen drug, or an orchiectomy (removal of the testicles).

The LHRH agonist drugs—leuprolide (Lupron) or goserlin (Zoladex)—shut down most of the body's production of testosterone; they are injected once every month, often for life. Like all hormone suppression therapies, they often cause hot flashes, loss of libido, breast enlargement, loss of muscle mass, and occasionally impotence. One drawback to the use of these LHRH agonist drugs is that they are extremely expensive.

Another drug usually used in combination with the LHRH agonists is flutamide, which is an anti-androgen drug which suppresses any remaining testosterone that the body produces. Flutamide works by attaching itself to prostate cancer cells in the same places that androgens would normally attach. Again, preventing the androgens from reaching the prostate cells will cause some, but not all, prostate cancer cells to die. Flutamide is generally taken orally three times a day.

The alternative option to the LHRH agonist drugs is orchiectomy, surgical removal of the testicles. This technique has been used since the 1940s for fighting advanced prostate cancer. The advent of the hormone suppressor drugs, however, means there is now a more acceptable option for most situations.

The Watch-and-Wait Option

The fourth option when diagnosed with prostate cancer is to do nothing except to have regular checkups. This is by far the most common option for stage A1 prostate cancers. The argument behind this therapy is the following: Many men who have stage A1 prostate cancer don't know it, live normal lives, and die of some other disease. Suppose you are diagnosed with prostate cancer: if it is a stage A1 cancer and you do nothing, you too will probably live a normal life and die of something else. So why go through the trauma of prostate cancer therapy, with all its unpleasant side effects?

Several studies have compared the life spans of men with early-stage, untreated prostate cancer with the life spans of men of the same age who do not have prostate cancer. Generally, little difference has been found. Studies have also compared the watch-and-wait option with radical prostatectomy, again for early-stage prostate cancers. No significant differences were seen between the survival rates in the group having surgery and in the group having no treatment at all. All of these studies, however, have involved small numbers of men.

Prostate Radiotherapy vs. Surgical Prostate Removal

Alongside the controversy in the area of breast cancer over mastectomy vs. lumpectomy plus radiation, the choice of treatment for prostate cancer represents one of the biggest controversies in the field of cancer therapy.

At its heart, the controversy between surgery (prostatectomy) and radiotherapy is about how to treat prostate cancers that are in stage A2 or B. As we will see, stage A1 cancers are now generally treated with a watch-and-wait approach, while stage C and D cancers are only rarely treated with surgery. Unlike the situation with breast cancer, however, there is a surprising lack of good studies in which the outcomes of these two options have been directly compared.

Given the lack of good trials in which the two treatments are directly compared, we have to make the best deductions we can from the evidence we have. It *appears* that long-term survival is about the same whichever treatment option is chosen. Specifically, about two-thirds of the men treated in the late 1970s for prostate cancer survived at least ten years, irrespective of whether they were treated with surgery or with radiotherapy.

So if the long-term survival is about the same, the real issue becomes the risk of complications from the two treatment options. Here, the comparison between surgery and radiotherapy becomes rather more complex. When complication rates are compared for patients treated at so-called "centers of excellence," such as major teaching hospitals, (see Chapter 8) the rates of complication are quite similar between radiotherapy and surgery. Surveys over the United States as a whole, however, reveal a very different story. Complication rates for radiotherapy are about the same for men treated at "centers of excellence" compared with the country as a whole. For patients who had undergone surgery, however, the recent nationwide studies of Medicare patients show complication rates are much worse in the country as a whole than at "centers of excellence." What this suggests is that the quality of prostate surgery is not very uniform across the country, and is higher in "centers of excellence" than on average.

In short, the best surgery is likely to give overall results comparable to radiotherapy for stage A2 and B cancers. "Average" surgery may give results that are not as good as radiotherapy.

In many ways, this apparent variation in the quality of prostate cancer treatment across the country is not surprising, because the prostatectomy is not a simple surgical procedure. Thomas Stamey, Professor and Chairman of the Department of Urology at Stanford University Hospital, recently wrote of the prostatectomy operation, "I do not know of any experienced surgeon who would not like to do their first 100 operations again."

Finally, one advantage surgery has over radiotherapy for prostate cancer is in terms of options if the initial treatment is not successful. If initial surgery is not successful, a course of radiotherapy is an option. If initial radiotherapy is not successful, however, the options are much more limited. Neither surgery nor a second course of radiotherapy is generally possible.

Prostate Cancer Treatment Options—Stage by Stage

In light of these considerations, let us see what the realistic options are, stage by stage.

Stage A1

In general the watch-and-wait option is the most appropriate. This is certainly true for the average man with prostate cancer, who is likely to be over seventy when the cancer is diagnosed. There is a point of view that younger men (under age seventy) should consider the same options as for stage B cancer (see below), in that the cancer may prove fatal, say, fifteen years later. The potential complications, in terms of incontinence and impotence, however, need to be carefully balanced, relative to very uncertain benefits.

Stage A2

For stage A2 prostate cancer, the watch-and-wait option is still one to consider carefully, particularly for older men or when the Gleason grade of the cancer is not very high. For men under seventy, however, the treatment options for stage B (surgery and radiotherapy, see below) become the most likely possibilities. As with stage A1, however, the potential complications of surgery or radiotherapy represent an argument for the watch-and-wait option.

At its heart, the real and difficult choice here is essentially between length of life and quality of life. If, at age seventy, you choose surgery or radiotherapy, you may well live longer, but you run a significant risk of suffering impotence (and incontinence after surgery) for the rest of your life. On the other hand, if, at age seventy, you choose the watch-and-wait option, you *might* live some time less than if you had chosen some active therapy, but you do not run an increased risk of living with impotence or incontinence.

The older you are and the lower your Gleason grade, the more the balance would seem to shift toward the watch-and-wait option. Ultimately, when all the facts and figures are digested, the choice between length of life and quality of life is the bottom line, and it is a very personal and difficult choice to make.

Overall, in 1990, two-thirds of all men with stage A prostate cancer chose the watch-and-wait option.

Stage B

Stage B is the most common stage of the disease, accounting for more than one-third of all prostate cancers. Stage B prostate cancer presents difficult choices between the three main options for treatment. In 1990, 41 percent of men with stage B cancer chose radiotherapy, 27 percent chose surgery, and 17 percent chose the watch-and-wait option.

Here, age and tumor grade must play a major role in the decision. A younger man, say, under seventy, with a low-grade (less aggressive) prostate cancer might well choose the watch-and-wait option. On the other hand, a man of the same age with a more aggressive tumor (say a Gleason score above 7) might choose to have treatment. In this case, because of the risk of complications and the extent of the disease, the choice between surgery and radiotherapy might weigh in favor of radiotherapy, unless a "center of excellence" for prostate cancer surgery is readily available.

For older men, say, above seventy, particularly if the cancer is a low Gleason grade, the balance may again shift toward the watch-and-wait option, because treatment may add very little to overall life expectancy, particularly if you are suffering from another serious illness.

Stage C

About one in eight prostate cancers are of stage C. These cancers are most commonly treated by radiotherapy. Apart from men who are quite elderly or who have another serious illness, this seems the most appropriate option. Surgery is generally not a good option for stage C prostate cancers. In practice, men who were found to have a stage C cancer during their prostatectomy surgery (in other words, the cancer was found to have spread beyond the edge of the prostate) often do well with radiotherapy after surgery.

If, for some reason, a curative treatment is not a practical option, then if treatment is needed for urinary symptoms, hormonal suppression therapy (see Chapter 4), sometimes with and sometimes without radiotherapy, is the most common option.

Stage D

About one in five prostate cancers are stage D, meaning that the cancer has spread to the lymph nodes, or further away in the body. Here surgery or radiotherapy is rarely a reasonable option, and hormonal suppression therapy (Lupron or Zoladex and flutamide, see above) is commonly used. For sexually active men, however, these drugs often result in a significant loss of libido, so the watch-and-wait option again becomes a reasonable alternative.

Lung Cancer

In 1994, about 172,000 people were diagnosed with lung cancer in the United States. While men still get lung cancer at twice the rate of women, the rate is slowly falling for men, but rapidly rising for women—a reflection of the increase in smoking by women and the decrease in smoking by men since World War II.

The lungs (see Fig. 6.5) are a pair of large spongelike organs whose main job is to bring oxygen into the body, through the air we breathe, and to remove waste gases from the body. Each

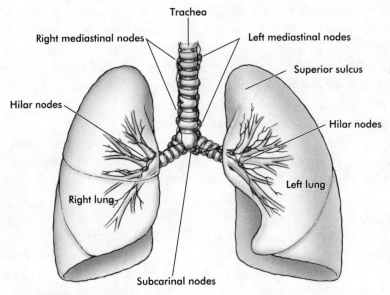

Figure 6.5 The lungs and the different lymph nodes that can be involved in lung cancer

lung is divided into sections, or lobes—two in the left lung, and three in the right lung. Essentially, the lungs consist of a huge network of tubes (called bronchi and bronchioles) through which these gases flow. The lungs virtually surround several other organs, including the heart and the esophagus, and contain many lymph nodes.

The most common first symptom of lung cancer is a persistent cough, or change in a previous pattern of coughing. A basic problem with diagnosing lung cancer is that there is so much space in the lungs the tumor can grow to an appreciable size before it causes any symptoms.

There are two different types of lung cancer: small-cell and non-small-cell lung cancer. In many ways they are entirely different cancers; they grow and spread differently, and they are treated differently. Non-small-cell lung cancer is by far the more common, by about three to one. Small-cell lung cancer, sometimes called oat-cell cancer, is a particularly fast-growing and fast-spreading cancer, rapidly spreading to other parts of the body.

Stages of Lung Cancer

Both types of lung cancer are categorized by stages, according to how far they have spread. Physicians use the TNM system (tumor, lymph node involvement, metastases), as with all cancers, but a simpler one-to-four system (I to IV) is usually used for non-small-cell lung cancer, and an even simpler two-stage system (limited stage and extensive stage) for small-cell lung cancer. Details of the stages are given in Table 6.3.

Treatment Options for Non-Small-Cell Lung Cancer

Stages I and II

For the more common non-small-cell lung cancer, when the cancer has not spread too far, surgery is the treatment of choice. Depending upon the extent of the cancer, the most common types of surgery are called the lobectomy (when a whole section, or lobe, of the lung is removed), and the pneumonectomy (when one of the lungs is entirely removed).

For patients with stages 0, I, and II non-small-cell lung cancer, however, there are occasional situations when surgery is not a practical option. For example, there may be some other

TABLE 6.3 Simplified Stages of Lung Cancer

	Tumor Size?	*Cancer In Lymph Nodes?*	*Metastases In Distant Parts of the Body?*
Stage 0	*In situ* cancer— very localized	No	No
Stage I	Tumor has not reached the chest wall, diaphragm, or heart	No	No
Stage II	Tumor has not reached as far as the edge of the lung, chest wall, diaphragm, or heart.	Tumor has reached the nearest lymph nodes	No
Stage IIIA	Tumor may have spread to the chest edge of the lung, chest wall, diaphragm, or heart	Tumor may have reached more distant lymph nodes in the lung	No
Stage IIIB	Tumor may have spread outside the lung.	Tumor may have reached lymph nodes in the opposite lung	No
Stage IV	Any sized tumor	Likely	Yes

medical condition, such as a heart condition, which makes surgery impractical, or the person may simply not want to undergo a major operation. Another possible situation is that after surgery begins the surgeon finds it is not possible to remove all the tumor. In these situations, for stages 0, I, and II non-small-cell lung cancer, radiotherapy becomes the next most practical option. Typically, radiotherapy involves daily treatments (excluding weekends) for about six weeks (up to seven or eight weeks for very aggressive treatment).

There is considerable debate about radiation as an adjuvant (additional) treatment after surgery for stage II non-small-cell lung cancer. In most situations, the added radiation treatment does not appear to improve survival. However, when examination of the tumor removed during surgery shows cancer cells right at the edge of the tissue that has been removed, additional radiotherapy is potentially beneficial. The idea is that if there are cancer cells at the edge of the surgically removed tissue (technically called *positive surgical margins*), then there are likely to be cancer cells remaining near the site of the tumor, and these cells would be killed by additional radiation. This adjuvant radiotherapy does not need to be as aggressive as radiotherapy treatment when no surgery is done, because there are probably a relatively small number of cancer cells remaining, so a five-week course is typically given.

Stage IIIA

Stage III non-small-cell lung cancers are usually divided into operable cancers (stage IIIA) and inoperable cancers (stage IIIB). Stage IIIA tumors have either spread into the wall of the chest, or to more distant lymph nodes, or both. As we have seen, the spread of cancer to the lymph nodes is a concern, because from there, cancer cells can move to other distant parts of the body, traveling through the lymphatic system. In fact, about half of all lung cancer patients have cancer in some lymph nodes. This is a reflection of the fact that cancers can grow for quite a long time in the lung without causing any symptoms.

If the cancer has spread to the chest wall but not the mediastinal lymph nodes, then surgery is the most common option, assuming that it appears possible to remove all of the tumor. As with stage II lung cancer, if it appears the edges of the removed tissue contain cancer cells, then radiotherapy is a reasonable option.

If the cancer has spread to the mediastinal lymph nodes, surgery is usually not possible. If surgery is possible—usually when the lymph nodes have been affected only slightly—then radiotherapy is an advisable option after the surgery. When surgery is not possible, which is usually the case, then radiotherapy is the most commonly used alternative option. Other alternatives, such as chemotherapy plus radiotherapy, have also been tried but the potential benefits may be quite small, and need to be weighed against the increased side effects from such intensive therapy.

About one in thirty small-cell lung cancers is a type called *superior sulcus* lung cancer. It is located at the top of the lung and often presses on nearby nerves, causing pain in the upper chest, shoulders, or arms. This cancer can be quite successfully treated with radiotherapy, usually followed by surgery to remove any remaining tumor.

Stage IIIB

In stage IIIB non-small-cell lung cancer, lymph nodes that are quite distant from the main tumor contain cancerous cells. This makes the tumor inoperable and, realistically, only palliative treatment to reduce discomfort, rather than curative treatment, is possible. A nonaggressive course of radiotherapy is the most common option for palliative treatment.

Stage IV

In stage IV non-small-cell lung cancer, metastases have spread beyond the lung. As with stage IIIB cancers, only palliative, rather than curative, treatment is possible, either with radiotherapy or with chemotherapy. Particularly in elderly people, the potential gains of these therapies, in terms of decreasing the symptoms of the cancer, need to be balanced against the discomforts of the treatments themselves.

Superior Vena Cava Syndrome

About one in thirty lung cancer patients develop superior vena cava syndrome, in which the vena cava, the large vein that returns blood to the heart, gets squeezed by the cancer. This situation needs to be treated urgently. The usual appropriate treatment is radiotherapy, at first given with large daily radiation doses to make the tumor shrink rapidly. Once the tumor has shrunk and the pressure is taken off the vein, the radiotherapy can revert to a more standard treatment.

Small-Cell Lung Cancer

About one-quarter of all lung cancers are the small-cell type, sometimes referred to as oat-cell cancer. This is an exceedingly fast-growing tumor and, by the time of treatment, most people with small-cell lung cancer have metastases in distant parts of their body, especially the brain, liver, and the bones.

In general, because the disease is likely to have spread significantly by the time of treatment, surgery is not usually an option. Limited small-cell lung cancer, which has not spread beyond the lung and the nearby lymph nodes, is quite responsive to the combination of radiotherapy and chemotherapy.

Because small-cell lung cancer spreads so readily to the brain, there have been trials in which the brain is irradiated, even when no evidence of cancer is there. While such treatment must still be considered experimental, there is some evidence that this "prophylactic" radiotherapy can produce a significant improvement in survival. Perhaps more important, by decreasing the likelihood of metastases in the brain, this type of radiotherapy can significantly increase the quality of life for people who responded well to the treatment of their primary lung cancer.

When the small-cell lung cancer is more extensive—in other words, there are metastases at places quite distant from the lung—chemotherapy is the most appropriate treatment. Average survival time for extensive small-cell lung cancer is less than a year, however, so the most important consideration is to maintain the best quality of life during this period. Here radiotherapy does have a role as a palliative treatment.

Cancers of the Cervix and Endometrium

Together, gynecological cancers account for about one in eight of all women's cancers. The most common gynecological cancers are cancers of the uterus (endometrial cancer and cervical cancer) and ovarian cancer. We will not talk here about ovarian cancer, because radiation is rarely used in its treatment.

Cervical Cancer

The overall incidence of invasive cervical cancer has actually decreased over recent years. Increasing numbers of younger women are being diagnosed with the disease, however, mainly because of increased use by younger women of the Pap smear test for detecting cervical cancer.

The uterine cervix, to give it its full name, is the opening of the uterus, or womb, which connects the uterus to the vagina (see Fig. 6.6). In its early stages, cancer of the cervix tends not to produce any noticeable symptoms, so the Pap smear is really the only practical way to catch the disease early. As the cancer develops, it will usually produce irregular vaginal bleeding or discharges.

If there are suspicious signs, the next step is for a physician to closely examine the cervix more with a colposcope—basically, a tailor-made magnifying glass. Usually a CT scan (computerized tomography, see Chapter 3), an examination under anesthetic, and a biopsy are the next steps to diagnose and assess the cancer.

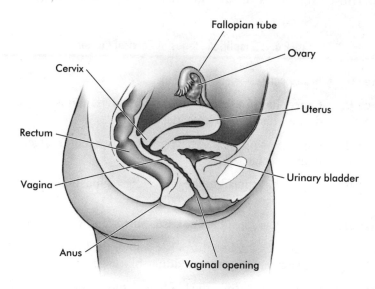

Figure 6.6 The cervix and surrounding organs

Stages of Cervical Cancer

As with all cancers, the choice of treatment for cervical cancer depends upon how advanced it is—its stage. While the TNM system (tumor size, lymph node involvement, metastases) as described in Chapter 3 is used to describe different stages of cervical cancer, a simpler system with a scale going from zero to four (0 to IV) is used more often in practice. The details of the stages are shown in Table 6.4.

Radiotherapy for Cervical Cancer

Radiotherapy is the most common treatment for cervical cancer. The treatment is usually given in a slightly different way

TABLE 6.4: Simplified Stages of Cervical Cancer

Stage 0	*In situ* cancer—very localized.
Stage IA	Cancer has not spread beyond the cervix, and is no deeper than ⅕"and no wider than ¼".
Stage IB	Cancer has not spread beyond the cervix, but is larger than for stage IA.
Stage IIA	Cancer has spread to the top of the vagina, but not to the tissue surrounding the cervix.
Stage IIB	Cancer has spread to the tissue surrounding the cervix.
Stage III	Cancer has reached the pelvic wall or the bottom part of the vagina, or is causing kidney blockage.
Stage IVA	Cancer has reached the bladder or the rectum.
Stage IVB	Metastases in distant parts of the body.

compared with other cancer sites, so we will briefly describe what happens.

Radiotherapy for cervical cancer is almost always given as a combination of external and internal radiotherapy (brachytherapy). Except for very early stage cancers, the external radiotherapy is usually targeted at the entire pelvic area, to try to kill any cancer cells that have spread beyond the cervix. On the other hand, the internal radiotherapy is more narrowly targeted on the cervical cancer itself.

External radiotherapy is usually given in daily doses (excluding weekends) over a period of about five weeks, with each treatment taking a few minutes. As with most external radiotherapy courses, this is normally done on an outpatient basis.

Internal radiotherapy (see Chapter 4) is normally done using a metal or plastic applicator containing radioactive material that gives out gamma rays. The applicator (see Fig. 6.7) generally consists of a central "finger" inserted into the uterus, and two sidepieces on either side that stay in the vagina.

Most internal radiotherapy to the cervix is done in two long sessions, one near the beginning of the external radiotherapy course, and one near the end. Each of these sessions takes about two days and requires an inpatient stay in hospital, because the applicator has to stay in place for the whole of the two-day treatment. In the past few years, however, there has been a trend toward "high-dose-rate" or HDR internal radiotherapy for cervical cancer, in which the treatment times are just a few minutes. Rather than two two-day treatments, this HDR internal radiotherapy consists of five to ten short treatments, done on an outpatient basis, with the applicator being removed between treatments. As far as is known, results of the conventional two-day internal radiotherapy and the newer HDR treatments are very similar.

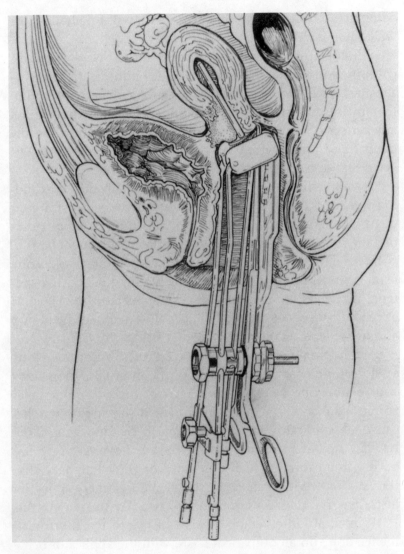

Figure 6.7 An applicator for internal radiotherapy of the cervix. Both the central "stem" which goes into the uterus, and the pieces at the base of the stem, which remain in the vagina at the entrance of the uterus, contain sources of radiation.

Treatment Options for Cervical Cancer

Stage 0 Cervical Cancer

Stage 0 cervical cancer is often called cervical carcinoma *in situ*, because the cancer has not spread from its initial site in the outermost layer of cells lining the cervix. This type of non-invasive cancer is entirely curable, either with cryosurgery (which freezes and kills cancer cells), diathermy (which heats and kills cancer cells), or laser surgery (which burns and kills cancer cells). Surgical treatment is also possible, although fairly unusual.

Stage IA Cervical Cancer

At this stage, a small amount of the cancer has spread deeper into the cervix, and surgery is by far the most common option. If the cancer has not spread too deeply, a minor surgical operation, called conization, is sometimes used in which a cone-shaped piece of tissue containing the cancer is removed from the cervix. This is particularly desirable for younger women who want to maintain their fertility.

If the tumor has spread more deeply, then a total abdominal hysterectomy is the next option, in which the uterus and cervix are removed. If the cancer has spread still more deeply, then a radical hysterectomy, in which the uterus, cervix, and part of the vagina are removed, as well as nearby lymph nodes in the pelvis is generally the most reasonable option. It is important to note that the ovaries are generally not removed, which is an important advantage for premenopausal women.

Stages IB and IIA Cervical Cancer

More than one-third of all invasive cervical cancers are either in stage IB or IIA, where the cancer has spread significantly in the cervix, and may have spread to the upper part of the vagina. Here there is a real and difficult choice to be made between the two options of radical hysterectomy and radiotherapy.

In practice, for these stages of cervical cancer, the choice is between a radical hysterectomy (with removal of some nearby lymph nodes), and combined external and internal radiotherapy. Results of past clinical trials clearly indicate that these two options are likely to lead to very similar results in terms of overall survival. So the choice really comes down to the question of side effects and overall quality of life.

Because both the bladder and the rectum are so close to the cervix, radiotherapy can cause side effects to both these organs. Rectal side effects tend to appear sometime in the first two years after radiotherapy, but bladder side effects can take as long as three or four years to appear. Roughly four patients in every hundred treated with radiotherapy for this stage of cervical cancer are likely to get serious side effects in the bladder or rectum. The corresponding complication rates after a radical hysterectomy are lower—about two patients in every hundred are likely to get severe urinary tract side effects.

An important question for most women with this stage of cervical cancer is the effect of the treatment on fertility, menopausal status, and sexual intercourse. In terms of the ability to conceive a child, it is possible to perform a hysterectomy and keep the ovaries intact, whereas radiotherapy will normally stop the functioning of the ovaries. In other words, radiotherapy will almost always bring on menopause in premenopausal women, who will normally then be prescribed some hormone replacement medication.

Perhaps a more relevant issue for most women with cervical cancer (who are already postmenopausal) is to choose the option that will have the least effect on enjoyment of sexual intercourse. Realistically, most women who have either surgery or radiotherapy for cervical cancer report that intercourse after treatment is less enjoyable than before treatment, in part for physical and in part for psychological reasons. Surveys on this subject suggest that somewhat more women who have had radiotherapy report sexual problems compared with women who have had surgery. The most common problem after radiotherapy for cervical cancer is a shortening or narrowing of the vagina, which can lead to discomfort or pain during intercourse. A vaginal dilator, however, can often help with this problem.

As well as the sexual problems associated with physical side effects of the cancer treatment, many women also report psychological problems related to the treatment, causing decreased sexual enjoyment. Because of this it is tremendously important to be comfortable with your choice of therapy, and perhaps more than with any other cancer, to involve your partner in the process of making that choice.

Stages IIB, III, and IVA Cervical Cancer

In these stages, the cancer has spread significantly outside the cervix, so surgery is rarely a practical option. Radiotherapy (and no other treatment) is by far the most common option for these stages of cervical cancer, and is considered the standard treatment. Chemotherapy has been studied in several trials as an additional treatment to the radiotherapy. This additional chemotherapy does seem to improve survival rates when used after radiotherapy for more advanced cancers (stages IIIB and IVA), and so would be a reasonable option for these stages. For less advanced cancers (stages IIB and IIIA), however, adding chemotherapy to the radiotherapy treatment does not seem to make much difference to the survival rate, and so is probably not a useful option.

Stage IVB Cervical Cancer

In this stage, the cancer has spread well away from the cervix, and the treatment is generally intended to be palliative, reducing pain, rather than curative. Radiotherapy is often used for stage IVB cervical cancers to shrink the main tumor in the cervix or other secondary tumors that might have spread to other parts of the body. Otherwise, a combination of chemotherapy drugs is the most common option. Whatever therapy is considered, the potential benefits of the treatment need to be weighed carefully against their inevitable side effects as the treatment is not meant to cure the cancer.

Endometrial Cancer

Endometrial cancer, sometimes called cancer of the uterus, is the most common of all gynecological cancers. About one in eight of all cancers in women are of the endometrium.

The endometrium is the surface lining of the uterus or womb, which is the hollow pear-shaped organ in which the fetus develops. Below the endometrium is a deeper layer called the *myometrium*. Unlike cancer of the cervix (the entrance to the womb), endometrial cancer often produces symptoms, in particular bleeding or discharges that happen at different times from normal menstruation.

If symptoms do occur, the standard test is called a D&C (dilation and curettage), in which the lining of the uterus is gently scraped to remove some cells, which can then be examined. A biopsy of the uterus is also done at this time. If the cells are cancerous, then a CT (computerized tomography) scan is usually the next step.

Stages and Grades of Endometrial Cancer

Like all cancers, the choice of optimal treatment is very dependent on the stage of the cancer (how far it has spread) and the grade of the cancer (how aggressive the cancer cells are). The different stages of endometrial cancer are shown in Table 6.5 ranging from stage 0 (least invasive) to stage IV (most invasive).

The choice of treatment for endometrial cancer also greatly depends upon the grade of the cancer—essentially how normal or abnormal they are. The scale here runs from grade 1, where almost all the cells appear normal, to grade 3, where most of the cells appear abnormal.

Radiotherapy for Endometrial Cancer

As we will see, hysterectomy (removal of the uterus) is the most common treatment for endometrial cancer. Radiotherapy, however, is often used either as an additional treatment or

TABLE 6.5: Simplified Stages of Endometrial Cancer

Stage 0	*In situ* cancer—very localized.
Stage I	The cancer is confined to the main part of the uterus and has not spread to the cervix.
Stage II	The cancer has spread to the cervix, but not beyond.
Stage III	The cancer has spread outside the uterus and cervix, but has not penetrated beyond the pelvis, or to the bladder or rectum.
Stage IV	The cancer has penetrated beyond the pelvis, or to the bladder, or to the rectum.

as the main treatment if there is some medical reason why a hysterectomy is not possible.

The techniques for radiotherapy for endometrial cancer are very similar to those for cervical cancer, described earlier in this chapter. As we shall see, however, often only external radiotherapy is given, whereas for cancer of the cervix, internal radiotherapy is almost always used, with or without external radiotherapy.

Treatment Options for Endometrial Cancer

Stage 0 Endometrial Cancer

Stage 0 endometrial cancer is often called *in situ* endometrial cancer, because the cancer has not spread from its original site, on the very surface of the uterus. If fertility is not an issue, then a hysterectomy is the treatment of choice. If future fertility is a concern, then a D&C (dilation and curettage) to scrape away the cancerous cells is likely to be as effective. If you choose the D&C option, then the hormone drug progesterone should be taken, basically as a precautionary measure. Progesterone can be injected or taken by mouth; its main side effects are weight gain and, occasionally, blood clotting, so it is generally not used if there is a family history of strokes.

Stage I Endometrial Cancer

About three-quarters of all invasive endometrial cancers are at stage I. In this stage, the cancer is either limited to the endometrium itself, or has spread only as far as the deeper levels of the uterus (the myometrium). The standard treatment is surgical removal (through an incision in the abdomen) of the uterus, both fallopian tubes, and both ovaries; technically this is called a total abdominal hysterectomy and bilateral salpingo-oophorectomy—usually abbreviated to TAH/BSO.

Whether radiotherapy should be added after the surgery depends greatly upon the stage and grade of the cancer. The idea behind the radiotherapy is to try to kill any cancer cells that might have escaped from the surgically-removed region or that are in nearby lymph nodes. If the cancer is not very aggressive (a grade 1 or 2) and has not spread to most of the deeper layers of the uterus (the myometrium), then radiotherapy is probably not needed.

On the other hand, if the cancer is aggressive (grade 3), or has spread to much of the deeper layers of the uterus, then radiotherapy is a good idea after surgery. Most commonly, external radiotherapy to the entire pelvis is used.

Stage II Endometrial Cancers

Stage II endometrial cancer, where the cancer has spread as far as the cervix, is quite rare. Only about one in twenty cases of invasive endometrial cancer are at this stage. Because the cancer has spread further and has often spread to nearby lymph nodes, radiotherapy is often given first, followed, after a break of a few weeks, by the same surgery (TAH/BSO) as used for stage I endometrial cancers. The presurgical radiotherapy is usually given as external radiotherapy over a six- to seven-week period, but giving the treatment as internal radiotherapy (or a combination of external and internal) is likely to be as effective.

Because so few women have stage II endometrial cancer, no large-scale trials have assessed whether radiotherapy is useful before surgery and which radiotherapy is best. The radiotherapy is essentially a safety precaution given in case some cancer cells have spread beyond the region where surgery is planned.

Stage III Endometrial Cancer

About one in ten women with invasive endometrial cancer have a stage III tumor, meaning that it has spread out of the uterus. If the cancer has spread only slightly outside the uterus, then surgery followed by radiotherapy is a reasonable option. Here the surgery would be a radical hysterectomy, removing the cervix, uterus, fallopian tubes, ovaries, and the upper part of the vagina. If the cancer has spread further, however, surgery is unlikely to be successful.

If surgery is not practical, a mixture of external and internal radiotherapy is generally the most appropriate option, as in stage II disease. If the cancer has spread to the lining of the abdomen (the peritoneum), then neither surgery nor radiotherapy is likely to be successful, and hormone therapy (progesterone) may be a reasonable option.

Stage IV Endometrial Cancer

About one in eight women with invasive endometrial cancer have stage IV disease, meaning that the cancer has spread to the bladder or the rectum, or outside the pelvis altogether. The most common treatment is a combination of internal and external radiotherapy, often with additional hormonal therapy. Generally, the goal with stage IV cancers is not to cure the disease, but to apply palliative therapy to reduce the size of the cancer and so reduce pain and bleeding.

Brain Tumors

Brain tumors are basically divided into two different types: *primary brain tumors* that start in the brain, and *metastatic brain tumors* that start in some other part of the body and migrate to the brain. About 17,000 new primary brain cancers are diagnosed in the United States each year along with approximately 150,000 metastatic brain tumors.

In fact, about one in four of all cancer patients will develop brain metastases at one time or another. The reason that brain metastases are so common is that cancer cells are carried in the blood to the brain, and then get trapped in the blood-flow system inside the brain.

The brain is a large spongy mass protected from the outside world by the skull (see Fig. 6.8). It controls all the senses, as well as memory, learning, and all muscular movement. Apart from the unique nature of the brain, what makes brain cancers very different from other types of cancer is the fact that the brain is completely enclosed inside the skull, so any growth in the brain is almost certain to end up increasing the pressure inside the skull.

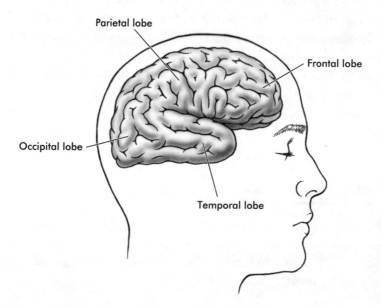

Figure 6.8 The different regions of the brain.

The most common early symptom of a brain tumor is a severe headache, particularly early in the morning. Other common symptoms are seizures, disorientation, and weakness in the arms or legs. Because different parts of the brain control different functions in the body, the symptoms of the cancer depend greatly upon where in the brain the tumor is located.

If a brain tumor is suspected, the next steps (see Chapter 3) are CT (computerized tomography) and MRI (magnetic resonance imaging) scans. After this, a biopsy needs to be done to remove a sample of tumor tissue. During this surgical biopsy, if the tumor is sufficiently small and accessible, an attempt is usually made to remove as much of the tumor as possible.

Malignant and Benign Brain Tumors

The first distinction between types of brain tumors is between *benign* tumors and *malignant* tumors. While there is no hard-and-fast distinction between these types, a benign tumor is generally not growing very quickly and is not likely to infiltrate to surrounding tissues. It is unfortunately true here that the term "benign" does not always mean harmless. If the benign tumor lump is not pressing on any vital part of the brain, it may well be harmless. On the other hand, malignant tumors are growing and have the potential to spread to other parts of the brain.

Types of Brain Cancers

There are a variety of types of brain cancers. Basically each type starts from a particular kind of normal brain cell, but for reasons we still don't understand, the cells start dividing and multiplying far more quickly than normal.

For all cancers other than brain cancer, we have been stressing how important it is to know the stage of the cancer, which tells you how far the cancer has spread. Brain cancers, on the other hand, rarely spread away from the brain or the spine, so stage is not as important in deciding on the best treatment. What *is* important for deciding on the most appropriate treatment is knowing what sort of brain cancer it is, and its grade, which describes how aggressively the cancer is growing.

By far the most common type of brain cancer is the *astrocytoma*, which originally grows from a star-shaped normal brain cell called an astrocyte. According to how aggressively the astrocytoma is growing, it is classified as either low-, mid-, or high-grade.

- *Low grade* or *benign* astrocytomas grow slowly but have a tendency to infiltrate into surrounding parts of the brain.
- *Mid-grade* astrocytomas, sometimes called *anaplastic astrocytomas*, grow faster and have a strong tendency to infiltrate to other parts of the brain.
- *High-grade* astrocytomas are the most common of all primary brain cancers. Sometimes called *glioblastoma multiforme*, this tumor tends to grow extremely rapidly and to infiltrate to other parts of the brain. High-grade astrocytomas also tend to produce a great deal of swelling in the brain.

Other than astrocytomas, the most common brain tumor is called a *meningioma*. Generally, this is a benign tumor that grows slowly and does not infiltrate to other parts of the brain. It can press on nearby parts of the brain, however, and so cause symptoms similar to those of a more malignant brain tumor.

Finally, as we discussed earlier, most brain cancers do not originate in the brain, but are secondary cancers having spread from some other original cancer site in the body. These are usually called metastatic cancers and often occur in several different sites in the brain.

Treatment Options for Brain Cancers

By far the most common options for brain cancers are surgery and radiotherapy, or a combination of the two. Generally speaking, if surgery is possible, it is the quickest way to remove a tumor in the brain or to reduce its size considerably. If surgery can be done without significantly damaging the surrounding healthy brain tissue, it is almost always the first option for brain tumors.

Some parts of the brain are inaccessible to surgery, and these must be treated only by radiotherapy without surgery. More common than either surgery alone or radiotherapy alone is a combination of surgery followed by radiotherapy. This is used in most advanced (high-grade) brain tumors, either because the surgery was unable to remove all of the tumor, or because the cancer has infiltrated to parts of the brain beyond where the surgery was performed.

Treatment Options for Low-Grade Astrocytomas

If the tumor is producing no neurological symptoms other than an occasional seizure, the watch-and-wait option is reasonable. As neurological symptoms start to develop, the first option for low-grade astrocytomas is surgery, with the aim of completely removing the tumor. Whether radiotherapy should be given as well depends very much on the results of the surgery. If the surgeon was able to entirely remove the tumor, then radiotherapy is probably not needed. On the other hand, in most cases, it is not possible to remove all the cancer during surgery because of the chance of doing too much damage to nearby healthy tissue. In this situation radiotherapy is a reasonable addition to the surgical treatment.

Treatment Options for Medium- and High-Grade Astrocytomas

Technically called anaplastic astrocytoma and glioblastoma multiforme, some of these cancer cells are very likely to have started to spread away from the location of the original cancer. Because of this likely spread, a two-pronged approach of surgery followed by radiotherapy is a significantly better option than surgery alone, and clearly improves survival rates.

There is also evidence that a three-pronged attack of surgery, followed by radiotherapy, followed by chemotherapy, is the most promising approach to get the best survival outcome. In particular, a "cocktail" of cancer-killing drugs known as PCV is showing a great deal of promise when used after surgery and radiotherapy, especially for medium-grade (anaplastic) astrocytomas. As with many multipronged treatment options involving chemotherapy, however, there is a significant risk of side effects for such an intensive treatment course.

Treatment Options for Meningiomas

The treatment options for benign meningiomas are much the same as for benign (low-grade) astrocytomas. Surgery is usually the first option, and if all the tumor can be removed, no further treatment is called for. On the other hand, if all the tumor could not be removed, then radiotherapy is a reasonable option after the surgery. Because the cancer is benign and growing slowly, there is no great urgency to have the radiotherapy. A reasonable option is to have regular examinations, and to defer the radiotherapy until there are signs the cancer has started growing again.

A new radiotherapy technique may well be a reasonable alternative to surgery for meningiomas. This is called *radiosurgery* or, sometimes, the *gamma knife*. The technique is described in more detail in Chapter 4. The technique applies computer technology to aim a series of very narrow beams of radiation at the tumor, each beam coming from a different direction. Particularly if the tumor is located in a part of the brain difficult to reach with surgery, this radiosurgery technique is very promising, requiring far less time in hospital than surgery.

While surgery is normally the first option for people with benign, slow-growing brain cancers, it is not necessary in every case. If the tumor is growing slowly and the symptoms of the cancer are tolerable, doing nothing at all is a very real option, particularly in older people.

Treatment Options for Brain Metastases

Brain metastases—secondary cancers from a tumor located elsewhere in the body—are by far the most common cancers in the brain. Radiotherapy is by far the most common treatment in these cases. The main goal of treatment is usually to reduce any symptoms caused by the brain tumor, and so to maintain a reasonable quality of life.

Because there might be more tumor cells in other parts of the brain, radiotherapy is usually given to the whole of the brain. It is given over a fairly short period of time, often two weeks. Steroid drugs may also be useful to reduce any swelling in the brain.

A drawback with radiotherapy treatment to the whole brain is that it can only be done once; healthy brain tissues cannot tolerate a second course of treatment. A promising new radiotherapy technique able to overcome this problem is the same one used for meningiomas—radiosurgery or the gamma knife. This radiotherapy technique (see Chapter 4) allows many narrow beams of radiation to be aimed at the tumor from many different directions. The result is that the tumor itself receives a large amount of radiation, whereas nearby healthy brain tissues receive a relatively small dose.

Head and Neck Cancers

Overall, there are about 42,000 new cases of cancers in the head and neck (excluding the brain) each year in the United States. About 12,000 of these are cancer of the larynx, and the remainder are various oral cancers, including cancer of the tongue, pharynx, lip, and various others.

Radiotherapy has a special place in the treatment of head and neck cancers. This is because the main alternative—surgery—can cause a loss of function (such as loss of voice in laryngeal cancer), or produce an undesirable cosmetic result.

We will focus here on three of the most common head and neck cancers: larynx, lip, and tongue. Together these make up almost half of all head and neck cancers.

Cancer of the Larynx

Cancer of the larynx, or voice box, is by far the most common cancer of the head and neck, representing about one-third of these cancers. About eight cases out of every ten are in men.

Like lung cancer, cancer of the larynx is strongly linked to smoking, and like lung cancer, the incidence of laryngeal cancer is rising in women.

The larynx, or voice box, is a triangular-shaped air passageway joining the pharynx (from above) with the windpipe (trachea) below (see Fig. 6.9). The larynx is designed to let air through, but not food. Its most important function is to contain the vocal cords, which vibrate to produce the sounds we make when we speak. The larynx is divided into three parts; the central part is the glottis, which contains the vocal cords. Above the glottis is the supraglottis, and below the glottis is the subglottis, which is attached to the windpipe.

Cancer of the larynx usually first shows itself as a persistent sore throat or hoarseness. A physician can examine the larynx

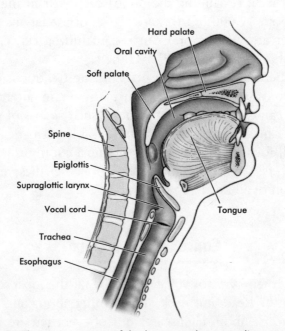

Figure 6.9. The various parts of the larynx and surrounding organs

with a laryngoscope, which shines a light directly onto the larynx, to look for abnormal lesions. Another test is to assess the flexibility of the vocal cords, by asking the patient to say "eee," which should normally bring the vocal cords together. If there is still cause for suspicion, the next step is a biopsy to remove some cells for examination.

As with all cancers, the best treatment option is generally related to the stage of the cancer. While the TNM staging system (see Chapter 3) is increasingly being used, laryngeal cancers are generally grouped into five stages (0 through IV), as described in Table 6.6.

Treatment Options for Cancers of the Larynx

In choosing between surgery and radiotherapy, the side effects of the treatment need to be considered. About one in five pa-

TABLE 6.6: Simplified Stages of Cancer of the Larynx

Stage 0	*In situ* cancer—very localized.
Stage I	Cancer has not spread from its original location. Vocal cords functioning normally.
Stage II	Cancer has spread to other parts of the larynx; vocal cords may be impaired.
Stage III	Glottic cancer has not spread beyond the larynx; supraglottic cancer may have spread just beyond the larynx. Vocal cords may be impaired. A small tumor may have been detected in one nearby lymph node.
Stage IV	Cancer may have spread beyond the larynx. Vocal cords may not be functioning. One or more tumors may have been detected in lymph nodes. Metastases may have developed in distant parts of the body.

tients undergoing surgery to the larynx have severe side effects, such as wound infection, fistulas, or damage to the carotid artery. About one in twenty patients undergoing radiotherapy have severe side effects.

In general, whenever possible, radiotherapy is the most desirable option for treating laryngeal cancer because it preserves the quality of the voice, as well as avoiding a major operation. Surgery can still be used as a second line of attack if the radiotherapy is not successful.

It is important to know that surgery does not always result in loss of the voice. In many situations, only part of the vocal cords are removed (hemilaryngectomy), or the vocal cords can be spared entirely (as, for example, in supraglottic laryngectomy). Nevertheless, radiotherapy is clearly a preferable option where possible, and voice quality is almost always better after radiotherapy than after "voice-sparing" surgery.

Stage I Laryngeal Cancer of the Glottis

Here the cancer has not spread beyond the vocal cords, which can still move normally. Radiotherapy and surgery both give very good results in terms of survival (about nine out of ten people survive more than five years with no recurrence of the disease), so radiotherapy becomes the more reasonable option, as it preserves voice quality.

Stage I Laryngeal Cancer of the Supraglottis

Here, the cancer has not spread beyond its original location in the supraglottis, and the vocal cords are still working normally. As with stage I glottic cancer, both surgery and radiotherapy produce about the same level of survival (about eight out of ten people survive more than five years with no recurrence of the disease), so radiotherapy is generally the preferred option.

Surgery here does not necessarily result in loss of the voice, as the vocal cords can be spared, but there are often major problems with the larynx after the surgical procedure.

Stage II Laryngeal Cancer of the Glottis

Here the cancer has spread from the glottis, either upward or downward; sometimes at this stage the vocal cords are also not functioning properly. If the vocal cords are not functioning properly (not "mobile"), radiotherapy is still the preferred treatment, but surgery does become an option. Choosing radiotherapy first, however, seems the most reasonable option because surgery is always possible at a later stage should the radiotherapy be unsuccessful.

Stage II Laryngeal Cancer of the Supraglottis

Here the cancer has spread to other parts of the supraglottis, or to the vocal cords, but the vocal cords are still functioning normally. Again, radiotherapy is the preferred option, with surgery as the backup should the radiotherapy not be successful. It is important to realize, however, that three out of ten patients will have some relapse, and the backup surgery is almost always total removal of the larynx, which is not a voice-sparing operation.

Stages III and IV Laryngeal Cancer of the Glottis and Supraglottis

For advanced cancers of the larynx, the most common option is total laryngectomy: complete surgical removal of the larynx. In many situations radiotherapy is given after the surgery if the surgeon has reason to suspect tumor cells still remain, either near the site of the surgery itself, or in nearby lymph nodes.

If the cancer is not too advanced, radiotherapy, with or without chemotherapy, is a significant option, with the clear advantage of voice preservation. An advantage of this option is that if there is a recurrence of the cancer in the larynx, surgery remains a possibility at a later time. If radiotherapy is the choice, it is critical you be examined very frequently after the treatment—perhaps every six weeks for several years.

Cancers of the Oral Cavity

In the United States there are about 20,000 new cases each year of cancers of the lip and mouth, or oral cavity. It is predominantly a male disease, with twice as many oral cancers in men as in women.

Clearly the mouth consists of many different organs, but in terms of cancer therapy, they share a lot of common features. The key, as always, is to try to cure or control the cancer, while keeping cosmetic changes or changes in function to a minimum.

Because the mouth does not have a great number of pain fibers, the most common early symptom of oral cancer is a lump, or "canker sore," that does not go away. In fact, these cancers are often first diagnosed during a trip to the dentist.

While there are many different types of oral cancer, the four most common are cancer of the tongue, cancer of the lip, cancer of the floor of the mouth, and cancer of the gums and palate. As with all cancers, one of the main factors involved in choosing the most appropriate treatment is the stage of cancer. All the oral cancers we will discuss have the same method of measuring the stages, which are listed in Table 6.7.

The two main treatments for oral cancer are surgery and radiotherapy. In many instances, if the cancer is very small and has not spread, it can be surgically removed without a cosmetic or function problem. In general, though, for most oral tumors that are

TABLE 6.7: Simplified Stages of Oral Cancer

Stage 0   *In situ* cancer—very localized.

Stage I   Cancer is no more than ³/₄" (2 cm) across.

Stage II   Cancer is between ³/₄" and 1¹/₂" (2 to 4 cm) across.

Stage III Cancer may be of any size. A small tumor may have been detected in a nearby lymph node.

Stage IV   Cancer may have spread beyond to other nearby tissues. One or more tumors may have been detected in lymph nodes. Metastases may have developed in distant parts of the body.

neither very small nor very large, radiotherapy and surgery are comparable options, and the treatment giving the best cosmetic and functional results would be the one to choose.

Cancer of the Tongue—Stages I and II

Cancer of the oral tongue (the front two-thirds of the tongue) is easily the most common oral cancer. Except for very small tumors that can be easily removed, radiotherapy is generally the most reasonable option, so that function and appearance of the tongue remain. The radiotherapy is generally done with a mixture of internal and external radiotherapy.

The internal radiotherapy (see Chapter 4) is generally done by surgically inserting a series of fine tubes into the tongue itself under general anesthesia. Tiny sources of radiation, either wires or pellets, are then placed in the tubes and left in place for periods of three to eight days. During this time, a plastic dental protector is usually worn to reduce the amount of radiation reaching the gums.

Very often, a mixture of internal and external radiotherapy is given. An advantage of this approach is that the lymph nodes in the neck can also be irradiated—and the neck lymph nodes are frequently danger areas through which the cancer begins to spread.

Cancer of the Tongue—Stages III and IV

These more advanced cancers are generally treated with surgery to remove the cancer. If necessary, nearby lymph nodes in the neck are removed if there is evidence the cancer has spread there. Surgery should, in most cases, be followed by external radiotherapy. In some cases, however, a combination of internal radiotherapy (brachytherapy) and external radiotherapy can be successful, an option that has obvious cosmetic advantages compared to surgery.

It is important to realize that this surgery is major and potentially very debilitating. If the cancer is a very advanced stage IV type, particularly with metastases in distant parts of the body, a palliative approach may be a more reasonable option. Here the aim is to use radiotherapy to shrink rather than eliminate the main cancer.

Cancer of the Lip—Stages I and II

Next to cancer of the tongue, cancer of the lip is the most common of the oral cancers. Nine out of ten cases of cancer of the lip are in men, and nine out of ten cases are in the lower lip. The two main treatment options, radiotherapy and surgery, both produce very high cure rates, so the choice really boils down to which treatment produces the best cosmetic result.

If the cancer is very small and can be easily removed with minor surgery, this is a good option. For larger stage I and stage II cancers, however, radiotherapy is generally the option producing the best cosmetic results.

If the cancer is not too extensive, external radiotherapy or internal radiotherapy (brachytherapy) is generally used, with a lead dental shield to protect the jaw and gums. For lip cancers that have begun to spread, a combination of internal and external radiotherapy is needed. As with cancer of the tongue, internal radiotherapy of the lip is done by surgically implanting into the lip, under anesthetic, a series of very fine tubes or catheters. Sources of radiation, either wires or pellets, are then put into the tubes and left in place for up to eight days, during which time the patient remains in hospital.

Cancer of the Lip—Stages III and IV

Radiotherapy works very well for early-stage lip cancers, and gives a very good cosmetic result. For advanced cancers, however, particularly when the cancer has spread to nearby lymph nodes, radiotherapy alone is likely to be less successful. Here a combination of surgery followed by external radiotherapy is a more reasonable approach, if the aim is to cure the cancer. On the other hand, the trauma of the surgery, and the need for subsequent reconstructive surgery, need to be carefully considered if curative therapy is not the aim

Chapter 7

What Can I Expect *During* and *After* My Radiotherapy?

The great majority of people having radiotherapy receive external radiotherapy. Here, a beam of radiation is directed into the body from an outside source; nothing is implanted into the body and nothing is inserted into a body cavity. Consequently, the treatment is painless. Once each external radiotherapy treatment is finished, there is no longer any radiation in your body—you are not radioactive in any way.

Once you have made the decision to go ahead with radiotherapy, your treatment will proceed through various steps. Let's look at these steps from start to finish.

Simulation

A week or so before the actual therapy begins, you will need to spend one or two hours in the radiation oncology department for a process called *simulation* (see Fig. 7.1). In this process, all of the exact details of your body shape, and the location of the

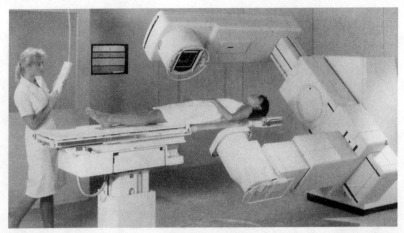

Figure 7.1 The simulator machine resembles the radiotherapy machine (see Fig. 4.1), but the aim here is to get precise details of your body shape and the location of the tumor so the actual treatment can be designed to be as exact as possible.

tumor, are recorded. The radiotherapy team needs this information in order to customize your particular treatment plan, so that as little radiation as possible is given to healthy normal tissues, and as much radiation as possible is given to the tumor.

The radiation oncologist and technician will place you in the exact position in which you will be treated—usually lying on a couch. It is important you keep as still as possible during each treatment, and so some kind of immobilization device will be custom-designed for you, which you will use during each treatment. For a patient with prostate cancer, this may take the form of a cast shaped to your body in which you lie during treatment; for a patient with head or neck cancer, it may take the form of a headrest or a mask or helmet. In each case, the aim is to make you sufficiently comfortable so that you can lie or sit without moving during the few minutes of treatment.

Now that you are in exactly the position you are going to be in during the actual radiotherapy, the next step in the simulation process is to take X rays, or CT (computerized tomography), or MRI (magnetic resonance imaging) scans. At this point the radiation therapist will make some dots on your skin (or occasionally on the body mold or cast) with semipermanent ink (see Fig. 7.2). These marks will be used to make sure you return to exactly the same position for each treatment.

Using the information gathered from the simulation and all

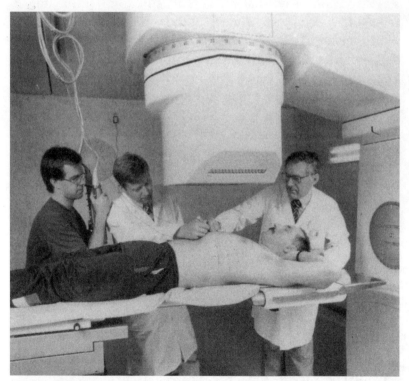

Figure 7.2 Placing the radiotherapy machine in the right position immediately before treatment. Marks on the skin are used to line up the machine.

the other tests you have had, the radiation oncologist will meet with the medical physicist and dosimetrist to plan the course of treatment: the total amount of radiation to be given, the number of treatments, the number of days per week, and so on. It generally takes several days for the calculations and planning to be completed, checked, and double-checked, and for any special custom-made gadgets to be fabricated.

For example, the radiation therapist may fabricate custom-designed radiation blocks or shields, which are put in front of the machine producing the radiation to block off any unnecessary exposure of normal tissue. This shield, or collimator, is made of a thick block of metal and has a hole cut in the middle to let the radiation through. This hole must be the same shape as the tumor, so it needs to be individually designed and built. Because you will probably be receiving radiation from three or four different directions, you will need a different collimator for each direction. These collimators are customized for you alone. They are labeled with your name and kept in the treatment room, ready to be mounted on the radiotherapy machine before your treatment.

Often, only one simulation session is required, but from time to time a second session is needed to refine the planning so that the best possible treatment can be designed.

The Daily Treatment

Your actual treatments will usually be given five days a week (every weekday) for a total of six or seven weeks. Some treatments are much shorter, lasting only two or three weeks, with only two or three treatments each week. Generally, external radiotherapy is done as an outpatient procedure, and most people go home between treatments and often carry on with their normal routine.

Before treatment is given you may need to change into a hospital gown or robe to allow easier access to the marked-up areas on your skin. It is best, therefore, to wear clothing easily removed and put on again.

The most common sources of radiation for external radiotherapy are called linear accelerators or cobalt machines. You will be given an appointment on one of these machines for the same time each day, five days a week. Usually, the machines are heavily used, and it is not unusual for forty patients to be assigned to each machine. Since they are complex pieces of equipment, it is also not uncommon for them to need some adjustment during the working day, and engineers are on call for this purpose. This can cause delays, so it is best not to schedule other important appointments too soon after your daily treatment.

Since the same patients tend to be treated at the same time every day, you may well get to know a group of people, scheduled before and after you, and a spirit of camaraderie tends to develop as experiences are related and stories swapped. Those who have been on treatment for some weeks can be an important psychological support to those just starting. There is much room for leadership and compassion here; helping others not infrequently takes your mind off your own problem.

Eventually it is your turn to be treated and the technician calls your name. Entering the room can be very intimidating at first; the walls are very thick, and the entrance is in the form of a mini-maze to avoid scattered radiation getting out. The center of the room is occupied by the linear accelerator or cobalt machine (see Fig. 4.1). The walls are often lined with rows of molds, helmets, masks, and collimators, each labeled with the name of a patient on treatment. As likely as not, some mis-guided psychologist, thinking to calm you down, will have had a large mural painted on one wall—suddenly you are on the beach in Cape Cod, or at a mountain lake in Colorado!

The actual treatment couch or chair will be exactly the same as the one you used during simulation. Your own customized mold, mask, or helmet labeled with your name is retrieved from the rows on the shelf and you settle down into position.

The technician then uses the marks on your skin to put the treatment machine in exactly the right position relative to you (see Fig. 7.2). The huge machine whirls up and down and ro-tates around you, until all is lined up. All is now ready, and the radiotherapy team will leave the room. You are on your own, or you think you are. In fact, you are being closely watched on closed-circuit television, and there is a micro-phone link so that the radiotherapy team can talk to you, and you to them.

Once you are alone, it is important to keep as still as possi-ble. Don't hold your breath—just breathe normally. After some period of silence, there will be a whirring noise as the machine comes on and generates the radiation beam; it will usually stay on for less than a minute, before there is silence again as the beam goes off. Within seconds, the technicians will be in the room to rotate the machine to a new position for treatment from another direction. This will be repeated three, four, or six times, according to the number of directions designed in your treatment plan. The whole thing takes only about fifteen to thirty minutes and you feel nothing.

Should you feel ill or uncomfortable at any time, don't hesi-tate to speak up; the machine can be stopped instantly. After the treatment is over you are done for the day, and you are helped off the table and back to the changing rooms. Then it's back home or back to work—but not before you touch base with your friends in the waiting room. They will want to know how you are feeling, and you will want a progress report from them.

At least once a week the routine is broken. Sometimes, after the treatment itself, X rays will be taken to make sure the beam is still lined up properly and aimed in the correct direction. Another simulation may be needed to change the treatment plan as the tumor shrinks. The nurse and radiation oncologist will want to talk to you, as will a dietitian, if you aren't maintaining your weight. Periodically, blood tests or X-ray examinations may be ordered to monitor your progress.

Internal Radiotherapy or Brachytherapy

Brachytherapy is so named because the radiation treatment is from a short distance away (*brachy* is the Greek word for short). It involves putting radioactive sources inside the body to irradiate the tumor—hence the name *internal radiation therapy*. Back in 1900, Alexander Graham Bell, the inventor of the telephone, first suggested that tumors could be treated using this technique.

Where internal radiotherapy is used, it often turns out to be particularly successful, but it is only suitable in cases where the cancer is easily accessible, either close to the skin or close to a body cavity. Overall, about one in twenty radiotherapy patients receive internal radiotherapy.

One advantage of internal radiation therapy is that the sources of radiation are placed close to the cancer, so that fewer healthy cells are irradiated. In this way a bigger dose can be given in a shorter time than with external beam radiotherapy. It is not unusual for a combination of internal and external treatment to be given. The internal radiotherapy delivers a large concentrated radiation dose to the primary tumor, while the external treatment delivers a lower dose to a larger region, just in case the cancer has started to spread.

There are two distinct forms of brachytherapy or internal radiation therapy, called intracavitary and interstitial. We will talk about each of these in turn.

Intracavitary Internal Radiotherapy

Intracavitary therapy refers to the technique of placing sealed radioactive sources into a body cavity close to and surrounding a tumor. By far the most common cancers treated this way are the female uterine cancers of the cervix and endometrium.

In this form of treatment (see Fig. 7.3), the tubes that will contain the radioactive sources, usually called an applicator, are put in place under general (or sometimes local) anesthetic. The actual radioactive sources are inserted later after you have returned to a private room. The applicator with the radioactive sources inside is usually kept in place for one or two days, and the treatment is usually repeated a second time after a period of one or two weeks. Intracavitary therapy is almost always combined with external radiotherapy.

During intracavitary internal radiotherapy you will need to stay in bed and not move around too much so the sources do not get moved out of position. Relatively large amounts of radioactivity are involved, therefore visitors are restricted for the one or two days that the implant is in place. Nursing staff, too, must keep their distance and minimize the time they are close to your bed.

Some institutions have devices, called remote afterloaders, allowing the sources to be removed from the patient into a lead safe each time a nurse enters the room. This means your everyday care can be carried out much more conveniently. However,

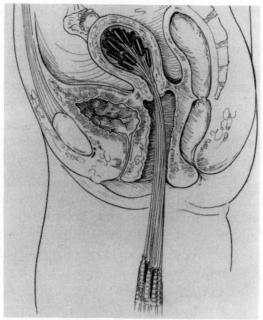

Figure 7.3 Intracavitary internal radiotherapy for cancer of the endometrium (see Chapter 6). Each of the tubes, which are inserted into the uterus, contain sources of radiation which irradiate the cancer.

the staff will take care to keep to a minimum the periods when the sources are in the safe (and not near the cancer).

There is no doubt that an intracavitary implant is not particularly pleasant. Generally, however, women get through the treatment without too much discomfort. If the applicator is causing you a lot of discomfort, do not hesitate to say so, and the radiation oncologist will prescribe some medication to reduce the pain and help you relax.

Usually at the end of the treatment the applicator can be removed fairly easily without anesthetic. Once the implant has been removed, there is no longer any radioactivity in your body, and you are free to receive visitors and leave the hospital when you are ready.

A recent development in intracavitary therapy is the use of high-dose-rate remote afterloaders. In this high-dose-rate treatment, the sources are inserted for just a few minutes at a time, under local anesthetic, on an outpatient basis. This procedure is repeated five or ten times over a period of about two weeks. Before each session, the applicator that will contain the radioactive sources is placed into the patient, and X rays are taken to make sure it is in the right position. The radiotherapy team then leave the room and the radioactive sources are transferred from a safe by remote control, through tubes and into the applicator.

The big advantage of this form of intracavitary therapy is that it avoids the need (and expense) of staying in hospital. Particularly for elderly patients with other medical problems, it avoids being confined to bed for a long period of time.

Interstitial Internal Radiotherapy

The second type of internal radiotherapy less commonly used than intracavitary radiotherapy, is called *interstitial* radiotherapy. Here, radioactive sources are surgically implanted, under anesthetic, directly into the tumor and the immediately surrounding tissue (see Fig. 7.4). The sources are thin, flexible wires left in place for several days (usually between four to eight days).

In some hospitals, a computer-controlled remote afterloader system is used where narrow tubes, called catheters, are surgically implanted into the tumor. After you have returned to your room, these tubes are attached to longer tubes at the other end of which are radioactive sources. When the treatment is ready to begin, the sources are shuttled along the tubes and into their correct position inside the tumor, all under computer control.

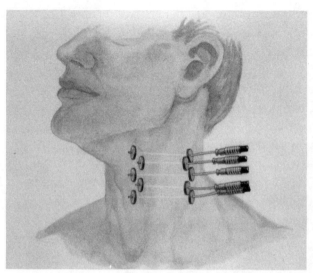

Figure 7.4 Interstitial internal radiotherapy for cancer of the neck. Tubes containing sources of radiation are surgically implanted in or next to the tumor so the cancer is exposed to a large dose of radiation.

The sources can also be shuttled away temporarily while the radiotherapy team or a visitor is in the room.

Except in institutions with a remote afterloader that can temporarily remove the radioactive sources, visitors must be very limited. This is because some of the radiation from the sources will escape from your body and will expose anyone else who is in the room. Generally, the radiotherapy team, especially the nurses, will work quickly and speak to you from the doorway rather than stand at the bedside. There also will be limits on visitors while you have an implant in place. Children younger than 18 or pregnant women should not visit at all. Visits should be brief and visitors should stay away from the bed. These restrictions on visitors need not apply if the sources can be temporarily removed into a remote afterloader, but still visits should be brief to limit the interruptions of the treatment.

Interstitial implants are particularly useful for treating head and neck cancers, as well as prostate, rectal, breast, skin, and bladder cancers. You are not likely to have much pain during implant therapy, but the radiotherapist can prescribe medication to help relieve any pain if needed. The anesthesia used during the original surgical implant may cause drowsiness or nausea, but this soon passes.

Usually, at the end of an interstitial radiotherapy treatment, the sources or catheters can be removed in your hospital room. Once the implant has been removed, there is no longer any radioactivity in your body, and you are free to receive visitors and to leave the hospital when you are ready.

Possible Side Effects of Radiotherapy

Because some healthy normal tissues are inevitably exposed to some level of radiation during the course of treatment, most people will have at least some side effects. By and large they tend to start a week or two after treatment begins, and subside within a few weeks after treatment ends.

There is quite a lot you can do to avoid or to minimize the side effects of radiotherapy. So it is important to talk about possible side effects with your radiotherapy team before the start of your treatment, and to take very seriously any suggestions they make. It is also important to keep your team informed if side effects do start. There are plenty of techniques and medications available that can ease your discomfort significantly.

We describe here the most common side effects from radiotherapy. Don't be alarmed. Almost no one gets all of them, but it is quite possible you will suffer from a few, hopefully in a reasonably mild form.

Tiredness

Probably the most common side effect of radiotherapy is tiredness. Of course tiredness is a very general term, but feelings of weariness, fatigue, or lack of energy are reported by most people undergoing radiotherapy. Generally, the feelings of tiredness are very closely tied to each radiotherapy treatment, and are at their worst a few hours after each treatment. For most people who are treated only on weekdays, the feelings of fatigue tend to get better over the weekend, during the two-day break from treatment. Generally, the feelings of tiredness start to go away after the radiotherapy course is finished, and are gone after a few weeks.

One of the best things you can do to ward off tiredness is to continue to eat and drink well. We will talk about diet later in this section.

Skin Soreness

During external radiotherapy, the radiation must pass through the skin on the way to the tumor, so it is not surprising that skin problems are one of the most common side effects of radiotherapy. Sometime after the first week of treatment, it is quite likely your skin will be sore. The symptoms are similar to a sunburn, and as with sunburn, fair-skinned people tend to get more severe reactions (though this is not always the case). This soreness will generally happen only in the area of skin actually exposed to the radiation. Areas of skin that are warm or moist tend to be the most sensitive to radiation, such as the underarm area, the area under the breast, and the perineum. Soreness almost always goes away within a week or so after treatment finishes, but the affected skin area might always be a little tender and tanned, and should always be well protected from the sun.

Many simple measures can help with skin soreness, much the same treatment as for sunburn.

- Regularly apply baby powder or cornstarch to the area being treated, as well as after every treatment.
- Don't wash with very hot water, and use a very mild soap.
- Don't use deodorants, perfumes, or aftershaves on the sore areas. Avoid shaving sore areas if possible.
- If the soreness becomes very bothersome, or the skin starts to get moist and ooze, your physician can prescribe various ointments, such as hydrocortisone.

Diarrhea or Nausea

The majority of people who get radiotherapy to the pelvic or abdominal region report some loose bowel movements or diarrhea. This tends to start a couple of weeks into the treatment, and generally goes away fairly soon after the course of treatment ends. Again, the best line of defense here is diet, as we will discuss below. A low-fiber, high-caloric diet is very helpful.

Apart from generic antidiarrhea drugs such as Kaopectate, Lomotil, paregoric, and Imodium, some specialized drugs have been shown to be useful in reducing the symptoms of diarrhea during and after radiotherapy. The two most common are called cholestyramine and sucralfate.

Mild nausea is also a common side effect of radiotherapy of the gastric areas. Again the best approach is through a reasonable diet, although it is a good idea not to eat for a couple of hours before the radiotherapy treatment. If the problem becomes severe, you should talk with your radiation oncologist about the new anti-emetic drugs proven to be very effective (if very expensive) in reducing radiation-induced nausea, such as ondansetron.

Hair Loss

If the radiation involves the brain or the head or neck, temporary hair loss (alopecia) is quite likely. Usually, this begins about three weeks after treatment starts, but the hair will begin to regrow about four to six weeks after the radiotherapy is completed. When it does regrow, it will not necessarily be the same color or texture as it was before. Hair loss is one of the more distressing cosmetic side effects of radiotherapy, but it is often unavoidable. Being prepared for it to happen does really help, and many people purchase a wig before starting treatment.

Oral Problems

For people receiving radiation to the head or neck, mouth and dental problems are quite common. The most common symptom is dry mouth and, less commonly, stomatitis, an inflammation of the tissues in the mouth. Dental decay is also often a problem.

The key to avoiding these symptoms as much as possible is to be very, very conscientious about oral and dental hygiene. You should use a mouth rinse at least six times each day, particularly after meals. Don't use commercial mouthwashes, but use a mixture of one tablespoon each of salt and baking soda in a quart of lukewarm water. As well as rinsing, this mixture can be very soothing if the inside of the mouth is sore.

Dental hygiene is also crucial. You should brush with a soft toothbrush and floss your teeth very thoroughly three times each day. Another useful approach to preventing dental decay is to apply fluoride directly to the teeth. The usual technique is to use custom-made dental plates soaked in a fluoride gel. These are held in the mouth for about five minutes each day.

Dental hygiene is important not only during radiotherapy, but needs to be taken seriously on a permanent basis afterward. Regular trips to the dentist are a must.

Most people treated for head and neck cancers develop some degree of dry mouth. This can be very bothersome. A drug called *salagen* may improve dry mouth considerably. If dry mouth is becoming a problem, talk to your radiation oncologist about using this drug.

Finally, sore throat, or difficulty in swallowing, can be a significant side effect for people having radiotherapy for head and neck cancers. Again, the right diet becomes the key here, and a liquid diet together with a mixture of aspirin and glycerin (aspirin mucilage) can often be the most comfortable for a while. Generally speaking, this soreness is largely gone by two to four weeks after the end of the treatment.

Loss of Appetite

Many people undergoing radiotherapy lose some weight—on average about ten pounds from start to finish. This is hardly surprising not only because of the radiotherapy, but also because of the stress, tiredness, possible pain, and changes in life-style that you are going through.

Probably the best thing you can do for yourself is, in combination with the radiotherapy team, to keep yourself well fed throughout the treatment. It is absolutely true that people who are eating well generally have fewer side effects from radiotherapy, and so cope better with the treatments. You need calories to see you through the treatment.

There is a superb free booklet (see Appendix D) called "Eating Hints: Recipes and Tips for Better Nutrition During Cancer Treatment," produced by the National Cancer Institute. It is well worth getting and following. In general, it is important to focus on eating, to choose foods you really like, and to make your meals a pleasant and special experience. A good breakfast is very important, as your appetite will often be at its best in the morning. Before dinner, an aperitif or a glass of wine may be a good idea, both to relax you and to stimulate your taste buds.

There is no need to limit yourself to eating at mealtimes—snack whenever you feel like it. Always keep a healthy snack available, wherever you are. If you find you are losing weight, drinking over-the-counter nutritional supplements between meals is a good idea.

When the Treatment Is Over

Once your radiotherapy treatments are completed, celebrate! You have completed the course. Bear in mind, however, that you have been through a tough time, so you should take it easy and continue to eat well and get plenty of rest.

More than likely, you will go back to your radiation oncologist for regular follow-up visits. If you had a combined treatment, probably you will also be scheduled to see the surgeon or the oncologist who prescribed chemotherapy.

These sessions will lay out your follow-up care, which will naturally depend upon the kind of cancer you had, and on other treatments you had or may need. You need to determine, with your physicians, how often to return for checkups.

Of course the most pressing question of all is, "How will I know if I'm cured of cancer?." The regular checkups will be one of the tools used to monitor your progress, but it is also very important to keep a close eye on yourself. Anything you think is odd or unusual needs to be discussed with your physician as soon as possible. A few specific areas to keep watch on are:

- Persistent pain in the same place
- Lumps or swelling
- Nausea, vomiting, diarrhea, or loss of appetite
- Significant weight loss beyond what you experienced during radiotherapy
- A fever or cough that doesn't go away
- Unusual rashes, bruises, or bleeding

Your early trips back to the physician will also help you decide how quickly you can return to the normal schedule of activities you had before the treatment. If appropriate, your job, diet, sexual activities, and sports are all areas you should discuss.

Most of the side effects of the radiation treatment should decrease significantly in the first few weeks after the radiotherapy has finished. You need to be patient over those few weeks, but if problems continue, discuss them with your physician. Plenty of medications are available to help alleviate the side effects.

It is important to keep looking after your skin. The care you were giving it during the treatment period should be kept up for several months after treatment ends. Continue to be gentle with your skin, and use mild soap and a moisturizer. You should be extremely careful about protecting your skin from the sun.

Chapter 8

Making the
Radiotherapy Decision

In this final chapter, we put together all the pieces of the puzzle, and try to guide you through the steps allowing you to make the best possible decision about radiotherapy. Specifically, we will talk about:

- The various types of oncologists, including the radiation oncologist
- Finding the right cancer treatment center for you
- Finding the right radiation oncologist for you
- Finding your own support team of family and friends
- Talking with your doctors
- Weighing the odds—making the radiotherapy decision

Finally, we will take you through a step-by-step approach toward reaching the best treatment decisions.

Types of Oncologists

Finding the right doctors is an essential part of the process of getting treated for cancer. So first, let us talk about what sort of doctors you may be dealing with.

The first distinction is between doctors who specialize in cancer and those who do not. More than likely, your primary physician—the first doctor you will have talked to—is someone broadly specializing in general or internal medicine. As soon as cancer becomes a possibility, however, you will be referred to an oncologist, a physician specializing in cancer treatment.

It is very important to realize there are basically three different types of oncologists who specialize in treating cancer in different ways. These are:

- *medical* oncologists (sometimes just called *oncologists*)
- *surgical* oncologists
- *radiation* oncologists

Medical oncologists specialize in treating cancer with drugs, usually chemotherapy. As the names imply, surgical oncologists treat cancer with surgery, and radiation oncologists treat cancer with radiotherapy. Your initial referral from your primary physician will almost always be to either a medical oncologist or a surgical oncologist. Either way, you will soon need to see a surgical oncologist, as you will need to have a biopsy (see Chapter 3) to confirm the diagnosis and help stage and grade the cancer.

At this stage, after having talked to a surgical oncologist and perhaps also a medical oncologist, many people decide on their treatment without ever having talked to a radiation oncologist. Ideally, your medical or surgical oncologist will suggest, before any decisions are made, that you speak to a radiation oncologist. This may not always happen, however, and if they do not suggest it, this is definitely the right moment for you to suggest talking to a radiation oncologist.

In a few cases, the response from your medical or surgical oncologist may be something like, "There is simply no role for

radiotherapy in the treatment of your particular cancer." As we
saw in Chapter 6, however, for many cancers there may well be
an option for radiotherapy, and this means you should speak
to a radiation oncologist.

Although it is certainly not always the case, it would hardly
be surprising if surgical oncologists have a general tendency
toward suggesting surgery, and if medical oncologists have a
general tendency toward suggesting chemotherapy. As we have
seen, in many situations there is clearly a best treatment option, and any oncologist will suggest that treatment, but there
are also many situations in which various options exist, each
of which has advantages and disadvantages. This is why it is
important to speak to a radiation oncologist, to make absolutely sure you are given all your options, in as balanced a
way as possible.

To see how the opinions of doctors can influence the treatment options that are presented to you, look at Figure 8.1. This

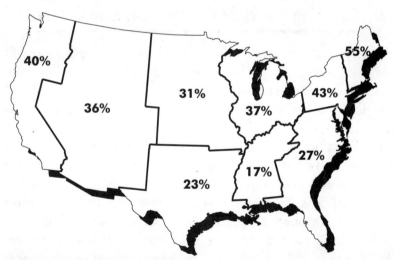

Figure 8.1: Percentage of women with breast cancer who have a lumpectomy plus radiotherapy.

shows the proportion of women with breast cancer who are treated with the breast-sparing option (lumpectomy plus radiation) in different parts of the United States. There is a huge variation across the country, from more than 50 percent in New England, to 17 percent in the Eastern South (Tennessee, Kentucky, Alabama, and Mississippi). What accounts for this huge variation? Of course there are a variety of reasons, but the main one is clearly that oncologists in New England are more willing to stress the recent trials (see Chapter 6) showing the breast-sparing option is as successful as the non-breast-sparing option. In other words, doctors' attitudes strongly determine what treatment options will be recommended to you.

The bottom line here is that we cannot stress too strongly the need to talk to a radiation oncologist, as well as your other oncologists. This will give you the best possible chance of ending up with a balanced view of all your treatment options.

Choosing the Right Cancer Treatment Center

After you have decided to see a radiation oncologist, you will be faced with the problem of deciding *which* radiation oncologist. Of course, the same applies to choosing your medical and surgical oncologist, so much of this section applies to choosing each of your oncologists. The decision about which radiation oncologist, in many cases, starts with a decision about which cancer treatment center, because radiation oncologists are often, though not always, affiliated with some cancer treatment center, often a hospital. So you may well choose a radiation oncologist through your choice of a cancer treatment center.

Let's look then at choosing the right cancer treatment center. The best advice is simple: Try to use the best facility that is practical for you to get to. Of course "best" is going to mean different things to different people, but we give some suggestions here. Specifically, we are going to talk about:

- Centers of Excellence for cancer treatment
- Comprehensive and Clinical Cancer Centers, designated by the National Cancer Institute
- Teaching hospitals
- Large hospitals vs. small hospitals
- Private radiotherapy treatment centers

Centers of Excellence for Cancer Treatment

Centers of Excellence are hospitals that have a national or an international reputation in the treatment of cancer. These hospitals have state-of-the-art technical facilities and, because of their reputation, tend to attract many of the best physicians. Of course, which hospitals fall into this category is a subjective call at best. We show a recent survey, whose results are very reasonable, from *U.S. News & World Report*, which ranks the top forty hospitals for cancer care, based on a variety of considerations (see Appendix A). Not all these hospitals are perfect, of course, but the odds are a little more in your favor if you can go to one of these centers.

Comprehensive and Clinical Cancer Centers, Designated by the National Cancer Institute

The United States National Cancer Institute (NCI), which is part of a federal agency set up under Richard Nixon's "War on Cancer," has designated twenty-seven cancer treatment centers as Comprehensive Cancer Centers (see Appendix B). To be a

Comprehensive Cancer Center is the highest accolade given by the NCI, and it only happens after a long and arduous review. The representatives of the NCI also revisit every few years to ensure that the high standards are being maintained. Comprehensive Cancer Centers are near the "top of the league" both in basic research on cancer prevention and cure, and also in clinical cancer treatment. They typically have teams of experts working together in research, teaching, and treating cancer patients.

As well as Comprehensive Cancer Centers, the NCI has designated thirteen Clinical Cancer Centers, which conduct both basic and clinical research (see Appendix C). These Clinical Cancer Centers also have been extensively reviewed by the NCI. Although they have not met all the criteria to qualify as comprehensive centers, they have been designated as providing state-of-the-art cancer therapy treatment.

As with the Centers of Excellence we talked about above (and some hospitals are on both these lists), not all the NCI-designated cancer centers are perfect, but you will stack the odds a little more in your favor if you can go to one of them.

One important word of warning here. There is no rule preventing *any* institution from calling itself a cancer center, a clinical cancer center, or even a comprehensive cancer center. The centers we have been talking about, and that we list in this book, are *National Cancer Institute-designated* cancer centers.

Teaching Hospitals

Teaching hospitals, where residents and interns and medical students are trained, have a reputation for being "good quality, but everyone comes and pokes at you all the time." To a great extent this is true. Generally, standards are high in a teaching hospital. Almost all of the top forty Centers of Excellence listed in Appendix A are teaching hospitals. Generally, too, the most modern treatments are more readily available in teaching hospitals. It is true, however, that you will be examined by a greater variety of staff in a teaching hospital, in addition to your own physicians. If you think this will be a major problem, then teaching hospitals may not be for you. If quality of care is the main consideration, however—and we think it should be—then teaching hospitals are an excellent option.

Large vs. Small Hospitals

In some ways, small hospitals—say, ones with fewer than a hundred beds—are very appealing. You can get more personal attention, and you are less likely to be treated as just a cog in a very big system. Bigger hospitals can be quite impersonal.

If, however, quality of care is the main issue—and we suggest it should be—then larger hospitals are generally preferable. Larger hospitals have bigger staffs, and so you are more likely to find oncologists specializing in your particular cancer. By and large, though it is not always true, larger hospitals will have more, and more up-to-date, equipment.

As an example of the difference between large and small hospitals, consider the statistics for breast cancer. In small hospitals treating fewer than 150 breast cancer cases each year, the proportion of women with breast cancer who receive the breast-sparing option (lumpectomy plus radiation) is only 25 percent (1991 figures). Contrast that with the corresponding figure for large hospitals treating more than a thousand breast cancer cases, where 38 percent receive the breast-sparing option.

Overall, while there are pluses and minuses to large hospitals, the advantages of a large hospital for cancer treatment are generally sufficient to make it worthwhile putting up with its impersonal features.

Private Radiotherapy Treatment Centers

Most centers providing radiotherapy treatment are hospital-based. This means, among other things, they have patient beds. In some states, however, there has been a trend toward independent, free-standing radiotherapy centers providing radiotherapy (and nothing else) on an outpatient basis.

It is hard to make general statements about these free-standing radiotherapy clinics. There are certainly some that are outstanding, but overall their quality is quite variable. If you wanted to play the odds, you would probably not go to one of these clinics, though some are undoubtedly excellent. If you do go to a private, free-standing radiotherapy clinic, a few questions to ask are:

- Does the facility have a full range of modern equipment, including linear accelerators, CT scanners, and internal radiotherapy (brachytherapy) facilities?
- Is there a full-time qualified medical physicist to take care of treatment planning and quality control?
- How many patients with cancers of your type have been treated at the facility in the last year?
- Are the radiation oncologists associated with a major hospital or medical center?

The Location of Your Cancer Treatment Facility

Of course, your choice of the best cancer treatment facility for you has to be a balance between the factors that we have just discussed and convenience in terms of location. Typical radiotherapy treatment courses involve daily treatments for up to two months. So location must factor into your decision, and you need to strike a balance in your choice to get to the best treatment facility that is practical for you.

To summarize, if you can afford the cost and inconvenience of travel, find the nearest major facility specializing in the treatment of the type of cancer you have. If at all possible, stay close to home so that you can enjoy the support of family and friends during therapy, and perhaps even continue to work. But don't jeopardize the quality of your treatment.

Choosing the Right Radiation Oncologist

As with every profession, most radiation oncologists are pretty good at what they do, some are outstanding, and a few are not so good. The question is how to figure out which is which.

The short answer is you really can't. What you can do is to stack the odds in your favor by choosing a radiation oncologist who works for, or is affiliated with, a top-quality cancer treatment center. This is why, in the last section, we discussed how to choose the best cancer treatment center.

Let us suppose now that you have tentatively identified a radiation oncologist, either by referral through one of your other oncologists, through your chosen cancer treatment center, or some other way. The next thing you can do to stack the odds in your favor is to make sure he or she is well trained and experienced in treating your particular cancer. You might reasonably ask:

- Is he or she board certified in radiation oncology (see Chapter 5)?
- Is he or she a member of the American Society for Therapeutic Radiology and Oncology (ASTRO)?
- Does he or she attend professional meetings for radiation

oncologists (such as the ASTRO annual meeting) on a regular basis?

- In what particular types of cancer does he or she specialize? (If you have breast cancer, you may not choose to be treated by the world's expert on prostate cancer, for example.)

More and more people now have medical insurance through health maintenance organizations (HMOs) and preferred provider organizations (PPOs). Clearly, the "managed care" approach of such health plans can limit your options when you are selecting your physician and your health-care facility. In practice, most physicians are members of one or more physician networks, and it is likely your HMO or PPO will have a wide range of oncologists available.

It is important to realize, however, that you still have options under almost all managed care plans. If your HMO or PPO does not include the oncologists you think you need, it is right and proper that you negotiate with them to allow you to use a physician outside of their network. Most oncologists are willing to see you under the fee arrangement set by your managed care plan. Many, and probably most, managed care plans are willing to negotiate this issue with you and to work with you to make sure you are comfortable with the doctors you choose.

We talk below about how important it is to get a second, or even a third opinion. Many managed care plans cover the expenses of such consultations. Even if they do not, they will almost certainly be willing to negotiate with you so that you get the consultations you feel you need.

Finally, if you start with one doctor and then find, for whatever reason, you are not comfortable with him or her, don't be afraid to change. Don't stay with an oncologist just to protect his or her feelings, or for any other reason. You have an absolute right to go elsewhere until you find the doctor-patient relationship that makes you comfortable.

Finding Your Own Support Team

Family and Friends

The day you learn your diagnosis is cancer is likely to be one of the most significant moments in your life. The news is traumatic, to say the least, and often hard to handle. For most people, it is important to share the news with immediate family or close friends.

Cancer does not affect the individual only, but the whole family. This is particularly true when the person diagnosed with cancer is the primary breadwinner or the principal homemaker—but in one way or another it is always true. Your disease is likely to disrupt your own lifestyle, and may well affect your family as much as yourself. Their support is very important as you face a serious condition. Plans are changed, prospects altered. The financial state of your family may be jeopardized, projections for retirement revised, work hours or leisure time modified. The life of everyone in the family will be impacted, and so they should participate in the discussions and in the major decisions.

Support from Outside the Family

It almost always helps to "talk about it." What seems like an intolerable burden, an impossible worry, becomes manageable when we realize we are not alone—others have walked this path before and many others face the same situation now. Look around any public room, a bus across town, a subway car; if there are more than half a dozen adults there, the chances are that at least one other person has cancer. In a group of older people the proportion will be even higher. Between one in four and one in five people in the U.S. population will develop cancer, mostly in their later years.

Some people, for whatever reason, choose to keep their medical problems very private. But for most people, a trouble shared is a trouble halved. Many support groups exist for people with cancer (some are listed in Appendix D), and most can be reached through the American Cancer Society or through your own radiation oncology team. A particularly strong camaraderie has developed among women with breast cancer, in groups such as One in Nine, and among men with prostate cancer, such as We Are Us. Some of these groups go beyond support for one another and play an active (and highly successful) role in campaigning for more research funds for their particular disease. But their principal purpose and reason for existence is mutual support. It helps to meet people with a problem similar to your own. When symptoms appear, you will be less frightened if you have been warned ahead of time by someone who has walked this path before.

Perhaps the best way of really understanding what to expect during treatment, whether it be surgery, radiation therapy, or chemotherapy, is through talking to other people who have gone through the same treatment. And remember, a fellow patient will probably have more sympathy, empathy, and feeling for you than your doctor or nurse can possibly have—however empathetic they are.

Do consider, however, that support groups in many respects are like any volunteer organization in that you get out of them only in proportion to what you put in. If you go to group meetings feeling sorry for yourself and assuming only that someone else is going to help you, it is not likely to be a useful or rewarding experience. These support groups are most successful when they have a core of people willing both to help and to be helped. Sharing is a two-way street.

Talking with Your Radiation Oncologist

Developing a good relationship between you and your oncologists, including your radiation oncologist, is one of the best ways of stacking the odds in your favor. Finding the best treatment requires a good relationship between you and your doctors. As in all relationships, effective communication is essential to developing this relationship. If you and your oncologist can get on the same wavelength about sharing information, evaluating choices, or participating in self-help groups, you are well on the road to getting the best treatment available.

Before talking to your oncologist, it is important to be clear in your own mind how much information you would like. Not everyone wants to know everything that's going on in their treatment, and not everyone wants to participate actively in arriving at a treatment decision. In fact, surveys have shown that nearly half of all cancer patients would rather simply be told what treatment to have, without participating in the decisions at all. Because you are reading this book, however, you probably do want to get involved in evaluating your treatment options.

During the first days or weeks after your cancer diagnosis, you are naturally likely to be very anxious in your discussions with your oncologists. However good the level of communication is between yourself and your oncologist, you may not hear or remember all that is being said. So it is useful, and certainly not impolite, to take notes, or to ask if you can tape-record your discussions. Never be embarrassed to say you haven't followed what was being said. Take your time, and keep asking until you do understand. And remember that there's really no such thing in this situation as a dumb question—if it is of concern to you it is not dumb.

Another good option is to bring a close relative or friend to listen in, to remind you of the questions you wanted to ask, and to help you recall later what was said. Having someone with you also helps share the information about your cancer, so your partner can better understand and help with decisions.

Before your meeting with your oncologists, it is often a good idea to spend a little time planning for the meeting. You need to think about:

- What you need to tell the radiation oncologist about your current condition, or changes in your condition.
- What you would like to ask the oncologist about your treatment options, or the treatment itself.

It is a good idea to jot down beforehand on a piece of paper what you would like to cover in these categories.

Weighing the Odds and Making the Choice

Every day of our lives we make choices, some in trivial things that are soon forgotten, and some concerning issues that will affect our lives for years to come. In every case, consciously or subconsciously, we weigh the odds before we make the choice. First, we sum up the pros and cons of the alternatives, the good news and the bad news. Then we choose the alternative we think has the most going for it. Choosing one option almost always involves rejecting something else. All of the chapters in this book have been providing information and background material to make it possible to weigh the odds in an intelligent and informed way.

As we have discussed before, in some situations there is little doubt about the best course of treatment. Obviously, making the treatment decision is easy in such a situation. Let's focus here on the common, but more difficult, situations, where there is no absolutely clear answer, since the different options give similar long-term survival rates.

Perhaps the most common decision to be made is radiotherapy versus surgery. Examples where this is a very real decision to be made are for early-stage breast cancer (the breast-sparing lumpectomy plus radiation versus the non-breast-sparing modified radical mastectomy), prostate cancer, and cancers of the head and neck. If the actual success rates of the treatments are virtually the same, then other factors have to enter into the decision-making process. To summarize the issues, typical advantages of radiotherapy are:

- No need for surgery and no general anesthetic.
- A generally good cosmetic outcome—no disfigurement and no loss of body functions.
- Treatment (mostly) as an outpatient with minimal disruption of lifestyle.

Drawbacks to radiotherapy include:

- A general fear of radiation.
- Concern about the side effects of radiation.
- The psychological disadvantage that the cancer is "still there"; it was not surgically removed.

As an example, in a recent study, women who were in the process of making their decision between the breast-sparing option (lumpectomy plus radiation), and the non-breast-sparing option (modified radical mastectomy) reported feelings regarding radiotherapy such as: "Radiotherapy might make me sick"; or "With radiotherapy the cancer might come back"; or "With surgery, I may look hideous, but I'll be cured."

While all these thoughts should be respected, they do not necessarily reflect the real-life situation in radiotherapy. As we have seen in Chapter 7, radiotherapy can have side effects, but they are usually temporary. Cancers do sometimes recur after radiotherapy, but they also sometimes recur after surgery—and we are talking here about situations where the long-term success rates for surgery and radiotherapy are about the same.

So really, if the long-term success rates for different types of therapy are the same, the deciding factor should be based on your own assessment of your future quality of life. And even when one treatment may have a slightly better long-term success rate than another, it is still important to weigh quality of life in the final balance.

Quality of Life

Quality of life is a very important consideration. What use is a treatment regimen if all it adds is a year or two of extra life filled with unhappiness, discomfort, and pain? For most people, extra months of life, bought by cancer therapy, must be productive and enjoyable to be worthwhile. Of course, "productive and enjoyable" will mean different things to different people. For some, just living is all that matters. For some, the ability to continue to work is the vital difference to a worthwhile life. For some, an active sex life ranks high in making life worthwhile, whereas to others it may be of secondary importance. No one wants to be encumbered with bags and bottles, pads and diapers, because of damage to vital organs, if this can possibly be avoided. The same can be said of physical disfigurement, loss of limbs, and loss of functions such as speech, sight, and hearing.

Remember, your cancer therapy itself may include a price tag in terms of pain or discomfort, certainly in terms of inconvenience and an alteration in life-style. There must, therefore, be a comparable payback in terms of enjoyable and productive life. Quality of life must never be forgotten in making your treatment choices.

A Step-by-Step Approach to Making the Radiotherapy Decision

Finally you have come face to face with your diagnosis of cancer. Here we summarize the seven steps that can lead you to your best possible treatment option. Follow them and you will give yourself the peace of mind of knowing you have done the best you can to stack the odds in your favor.

Step 1.

Share your problem with your immediate family and/or close friends. You need support and comfort from day one; you can often draw on the strength of others when you feel weakness in yourself.

Step 2.

Start reading and learning. Learn all you can about your condition, your treatment options, and your outlook. If you've got this far in this book you have made a good start. It is amazing and gratifying how much nonmedical people now know about medicine. For many, the days of blind faith in the "expert" are gone.

Step 3.

Choose your cancer treatment facility. If it is practical, find the nearest major cancer treatment facility specializing in the treatment of the type of cancer you have. Stay close to home if possible, but the quality of your treatment should ideally be your overriding consideration.

Step 4.

Choose a medical oncologist, a surgical oncologist, and a radiation oncologist. Make sure each is qualified, that they talk to each other, and ideally, that they are experienced in treating your particular cancer. Talk to them all, preferably with a friend or family member present, and preferably more than once.

Step 5.

Get a second and, if you wish, a third opinion. This is your best "insurance policy" against getting any sort of biased advice from your primary oncologists.

Step 6.

Weigh your options, bearing in mind the long-term success rates for your different options, and, crucially, the likely outcomes in terms of your quality of life. It should be your personal assessment of the balance between these two factors that ultimately drives your treatment decision.

Step 7.

The decision is yours. You have assembled your team of medical supporters, and friend and family supporters. Use them all, but make the decision that makes *you* feel the most comfortable.

Knowledge is powerful medicine!

Appendix A

Centers of Excellence for Cancer Treatment

The following table shows ratings of forty large cancer treatment centers, taken from a physicians' survey reported in *U.S. News and World Report.* The ratings are for cancer treatment in general, and not specifically for radiotherapy departments. The exact numbers do not mean much. It is important to recognize that patients were not consulted in this survey. Many other large centers probably deserve to be included, but the institutions on this list certainly merit being called "Center of Excellence."

APPENDIX A: Centers of Excellence for Cancer Treatment

Rank	Hospital	Overall Score	Reputation Score (out of 100)	Ratio of Interns/Residents to Beds	Technology Score (out of 12)	Ratio of R.N.s to Beds	Ratio of Board-Certified Oncologists to Beds
1	Memorial Sloan-Kettering Cancer Center, New York City	100	70.8	0.38	9	1.37	0.08
2	M. D. Anderson Cancer Center, Houston	93.2	63.1	0.70	11	1.88	0.01
3	Dana-Farber Cancer Institute, Boston	74.1	46.7	0.49	4	1.58	0.96
4	Johns Hopkins Hospital, Baltimore	47.7	28.7	0.73	11	1.43	0.01
5	Mayo Clinic, Rochester, Minn.	42.3	27.5	0.24	8	0.77	0.03
6	Stanford University Hospital, Stanford, Calif.	30.9	15.3	1.34	10	0.86	0.03
7	University of Washington Medical Center, Seattle	30.7	13.1	1.05	9	2.06	0.04
8	Duke University Medical Center, Durham, N.C.	28.7	12.3	0.91	12	1.6	0.03
9	University of Chicago Hospitals	25.1	8.1	1.64	11	1.38	0.03

Source: *U.S. News & World Report,* July 24, 1995

Rank	Hospital	Overall Score	Reputation Score (out of 100)	Ratio of Interns/Residents to Beds	Technology Score (out of 12)	Ratio of R.N.s to Beds	Ratio of Board-Certified Oncologists to Beds
10	Roswell Park Cancer Institute, Buffalo	24.7	8.5	0.68	9	2.58	0.00
11	University of California, San Francisco	21.2	6.0	1.03	11	1.82	0.02
12	Massachusetts General Hospital, Boston	21.1	7.3	1.00	12	1.14	0.01
13	UCLA Medical Center, Los Angeles	19.4	4.4	1.52	11	1.20	0.03
14	University of Pennsylvania Hospital, Philadelphia	19.2	4.0	1.72	10	1.33	0.03
15	University of California, Davis Medical Center	19.2	0.8	1.54	11	2.81	0.02
16	Indiana University Medical Center, Indianapolis	18.4	3.4	1.10	11	1.86	0.02
17	UCSD Medical Center, San Diego	16.8	0.4	1.65	8	2.17	0.06
18	University Hospital, Portland, Ore.	16.2	0.0	1.54	9	2.31	0.02
19	Fox Chase Cancer Center, Philadelphia	16.1	3.7	0.36	7	1.42	0.29

Continued overleaf

APPENDIX A: Centers of Excellence for Cancer Treatment, continued

Rank	Hospital	Overall Score	Reputation Score (out of 100)	Ratio of Interns/Residents to Beds	Technology Score (out of 12)	Ratio of R.N.s to Beds	Ratio of Board-Certified Oncologists to Beds
20	University Medical Center, Tucson	15.9	3.0	0.74	9	1.73	0.05
21	University of Nebraska Medical Center, Omaha	15.9	2.8	1.37	10	1.23	0.00
22	University of Wisconsin Hospitals, Madison	15.8	2.0	1.30	11	1.24	0.04
23	Cleveland Clinic	15.8	1.9	1.22	11	1.47	0.01
24	Vanderbilt University Hospital, Nashville	15.6	1.9	1.21	12	1.29	0.01
25	University Hospitals of Cleveland	15.5	0.0	1.60	12	1.73	0.03
26	University of Pittsburgh-Presbyterian Hospital	15.5	0.0	1.48	8	2.10	0.06
27	University of Virginia, Charlottesville	15.3	0.0	1.41	11	1.92	0.01
28	F. G. McGaw Hospital at Loyola University, Illinois	15.1	0.4	1.46	11	1.59	0.03
29	Mount Sinai Medical Center, New York City	14.9	2.6	0.99	9	1.50	0.01

Rank	Hospital	Overall Score	Reputation Score (out of 100)	Ratio of Interns/Residents to Beds	Technology Score (out of 12)	Ratio of R.N.s to Beds	Ratio of Board-Certified Oncologists to Beds
30	University Hospitals, Oklahoma City	14.9	0.0	1.60	11	1.56	0.03
31	University of North Carolina Hospitals, Chapel Hill	14.3	0.6	1.41	10	1.71	0.01
32	Brigham and Women's Hospital, Boston	14.7	1.9	1.49	10	0.79	0.07
33	St. Louis University Hospital	14.7	0.0	1.89	10	1.33	0.02
34	University of Illinois Hospital and Clinics, Chicago	14.2	0.0	1.29	9	1.95	0.02
35	Henry Ford Hospital, Detroit	14.1	0.5	1.34	10	1.50	0.00
36	Yale-New Haven Hospital, New Haven, Conn.	14.1	1.3	1.12	10	1.23	0.04
37	USC Kenneth Norris Cancer Hospital, Los Angeles	14.0	1.3	0.40	8	1.37	0.40
38	Penn State, Hershey, Illinois	14.0	0.0	1.55	9	1.57	0.01
39	Barnes Hospital, St. Louis	13.9	2.7	0.89	11	0.82	0.00
40	University of Michigan Medical Center, Ann Arbor	13.9	1.6	1.00	10	1.29	0.01

Appendix B

NCI-Designated Comprehensive Cancer Centers

ALABAMA
University of Alabama at Birmingham
Comprehensive Cancer Center
1918 University Boulevard
Birmingham, AL 35294
(205) 934-5077

ARIZONA
University of Arizona Cancer Center
1501 North Campbell Avenue
Tucson, AZ 85724
(602) 626-6372

CALIFORNIA
USC/Norris Comprehensive Cancer Center
1441 Eastlake Avenue
Los Angeles, CA 90033-0804
(213) 226-2370

Jonsson Comprehensive Cancer Center
University of California at Los Angeles
100 UCLA Medical Plaza, Suite 255
Los Angeles, CA 90024-1781
(800) 825-2631

CONNECTICUT
Yale Cancer Center
Yale University School of Medicine
P.O. Box 208028
333 Cedar Street
New Haven, CT 06510-8028
(203) 785-4095

DISTRICT OF COLUMBIA
Lombardi Cancer Research Center
Georgetown University Medical Center
3800 Reservoir Road NW
Washington, DC 20007
(202) 687-2192

FLORIDA
Sylvester Comprehensive Cancer Center
University of Miami Medical School
1475 Northwest 12th Avenue
Miami, FL 33136
(305) 545-1000

MARYLAND
The Johns Hopkins Oncology Center
600 North Wolfe Street
Baltimore, MD 21287-8915
(410) 955-8964

MASSACHUSETTS
Dana-Farber Cancer Institute
44 Binney Street
Boston, MA 02115
(617) 632-3476

MICHIGAN
Meyer L. Prentis Comprehensive Cancer Center of
Metropolitan Detroit
110 East Warren Avenue
Detroit, MI 48201
(313) 745-4329

University of Michigan
Comprehensive Cancer Center
101 Simpson Drive
Ann Arbor, MI 48109-0752
(313) 936-9583

MINNESOTA
Mayo Comprehensive Cancer Center
200 First Street SW
Rochester, MN 55902
(507) 284-3413

NEW HAMPSHIRE
Norris Cotton Cancer Center
Dartmouth-Hitchcock Medical Center
2 Mynard Street
Hanover, NH 03756
(603) 646-5505

NEW YORK
Kaplan Cancer Center
New York University Medical Center
462 First Avenue
New York, NY 10016-9103
(212) 263-6485

Memorial Sloan-Kettering Cancer Center
1275 York Avenue
New York, NY 10021
(800) 525-2225

Roswell Park Cancer Institute
Elm and Carlton Streets
Buffalo, NY 14263
(800) 767-9355

NORTH CAROLINA
Duke Comprehensive Cancer Center
P.O. Box 3814
Durham, NC 27710
(919) 684-2748

UNC Lineberger Comprehensive Cancer Center
University of North Carolina School of Medicine
Chapel Hill, NC 27599
(919) 966-4431

Cancer Center of Wake Forest University at
Bowman Gray School of Medicine
300 South Hawthorne Road
Winston-Salem, NC 27103
(919)748-4354

OHIO
Ohio State University Comprehensive Cancer Center
Arthur G. James Cancer Hospital
410 West 10th Avenue
Columbus, OH 43210
(800) 638-6996

PENNSYLVANIA
Fox Chase Cancer Center
7701 Burholme Avenue
Philadelphia, PA 19111
(215) 728-2570

University of Pennsylvania Cancer Center
3400 Spruce Street
Philadelphia, PA 19104
(215) 662-6364

Pittsburgh Cancer Institute
200 Meyran Avenue
Pittsburgh, PA 15213-2592
(800) 537-4063

TEXAS
University of Texas
M. D. Anderson Cancer Center
1515 Holcombe Boulevard
Houston, TX 77030
(713) 792-3245

VERMONT
Vermont Regional Cancer Center
University of Vermont
1 South Prospect Street
Burlington, VT 05401
(802) 656-4580

WASHINGTON
Fred Hutchinson Cancer Research Center
1124 Columbia Street
Seattle, WA 98104
(206) 667-5000

WISCONSIN
University of Wisconsin Comprehensive Cancer Center
600 Highland Avenue
Madison, WI 53792
(608) 263-8090

NCI-Designated Clinical Cancer Centers

CALIFORNIA

City of Hope National Medical Center
Beckman Research Institute
1500 East Duarte Road
Duarte, CA 91010
(818) 359-8111

University of California at San Diego Cancer Center
225 Dickinson Street
San Diego, CA 92103
(619) 543-6178

COLORADO

University of Colorado Cancer Center
4200 East 9th Avenue
Denver, CO 80262
(303) 270-3007

ILLINOIS

Robert H. Lurie Cancer Center
Northwestern University
303 East Chicago Avenue
Olson Pavilion, Room 8250
Chicago, IL 60611
(312) 908-8400

University of Chicago Cancer Research Center
5841 South Maryland Avenue
Chicago, IL 60637
(312) 702-9200

NEW YORK

Albert Einstein College of Medicine
Cancer Research Center
Chanin Building
1300 Morris Park Avenue
Bronx, NY 10461
(718) 920-4826

Columbia University Cancer Center
College of Physicians and Surgeons
630 West 168th Street
New York, NY 10032
(212) 305-6905

University of Rochester Cancer Center
601 Elmwood Avenue
Box 704
Rochester, NY 14642
(716) 275-4911

OHIO
Ireland Cancer Center at Case Western Reserve University
University Hospitals of Cleveland
2074 Abington Road
Cleveland, OH 44106
(216) 844-5432

TENNESSEE
St. Jude Children's Research Hospital
332 North Lauderdale Street
Memphis, TN 38101-0318
(901) 522-0306

TEXAS
San Antonio Cancer Institute
4450 Medical Drive
San Antonio, TX 78229
(210) 616-5798

UTAH
Utah Cancer Center
University of Utah Medical Center
50 North Medical Drive
Salt Lake City, UT 84132
(801) 581-4048

VIRGINIA
Massey Cancer Center
Medical College of Virginia
1200 East Broad Street
Richmond, VA 23298
(804) 371-5116

Appendix D

Where to Get More Information

There is a wealth of further information available about can-cer and about radiotherapy. We hope that reading this book will have pointed you in the right direction, and we stress again that information will empower you, in collaboration with your physicians, to reach the best treatment options for *you*.

Books

The National Cancer Institute has a superb series of very brief books, all of which are free. We strongly recommend obtaining all of them. You can do this by calling NCI's Cancer Information Service, which we talk about more below, at (800) 422-6237. The books are:

- *Radiotherapy and You—A Guide to Self-Help During Treatment*
- *Chemotherapy and You—A Guide to Self-Help During Treatment*
- *Eating Hints: Recipes and Tips for Better Nutrition During Cancer Treatment*

- *Questions and Answers About Pain Control*
- *Taking Time: Support for People with Cancer and the People Who Care About Them*
- *What you Need to Know About Cancer* (This is a series of books about particular cancers—ask for the book about your type of cancer)

Two other short booklets that we recommend are:

- *Treating Cancer with Radiotherapy*, published by the American Society for Therapeutic Radiology and Oncology, 33 pages; call (800) 962-7876
- *Talking with Your Doctor*, published by the American Cancer Society, 6 pages; call (800) 227-2345

There are many good books about cancer. Just browse in your local bookstore. There are *not* many books specifically about radiotherapy. One we like is:

- *Coping with Radiation Therapy: A Ray of Hope*, by Dan C. Cukier, M.D., and Virginia McCullough (Lowell House, 1993)

Two more general books about cancer treatment and choices that we like are:

- *Everyone's Guide to Cancer Therapy*, by Malin Dollinger, Ernest Rosenbaum, and Greg Cable (Andrews & McMeel, 1994)
- *Choices*, by Marion Morra and Eve Potts (Avon Books, 1994)

Both these books contain a wealth of general information on all the different cancers and their staging and treatment.

These are excellent places to get basic background information on cancer.

Quite a few books on cancer have been written by survivors, who describe their experiences in trying to get informed, trying to come to the best treatment option, and then getting treated. Three that we like are:

- *If the President Had Cancer . . . Cancer Care: How to Find and Get the Best There Is*, by Gary Schine (Sandra Publications, 1994)
- *The Race is Run One Step at a Time*, by Nancy G. Brinker and Catherine McEvily Harris (Summit Publishing Group, 1995)
- *Prostate Cancer: Making Survival Decisions*, by Sylvan Meyer and Seymour Nash (University of Chicago Press, 1994)

Videos

The American College of Radiologists has produced a 23-minute video called *Radiation Oncology: Waging War on Cancer*. It includes interviews with the radiotherapy team, radiotherapy patients, and a look at radiotherapy equipment. It is available from the American College of Radiologists (800) 227-7762

Other Sources of Information About Cancer

Two very good sources of information when you have specific questions are the National Cancer Institute's Cancer Information and CancerFax services, and the American Cancer Society.

The Cancer Information Service

The Cancer Information Service (CIS) is a nationwide toll-free telephone service providing accurate, up-to-date information on cancer to patients and their families, health professionals, and the general public. CIS offices can be reached anywhere in the U.S. by dialing (800) 422-6237.

The CIS can provide specific information in understandable language about particular types of cancer as well as information on state-of-the-art care and the availability of clinical trials. The CIS also distributes free NCI books and pamphlets to callers (see *Books*, above).

The CIS staff work for the government's National Cancer Institute, and they have access to the latest information about current treatment, early detection, and supportive care. The CIS also provides referrals to cancer-related community resources such as support groups, smoking cessation programs, screening, hospice, home health care, and transportation services.

The CIS serves the entire United States and Puerto Rico. Hours of operation are Monday through Friday, 9 A.M. to 7 P.M., local time.

CancerFax

CancerFax is a free service provided by the National Cancer Institute enabling people to receive current cancer information through a fax machine. CancerFax provides summaries on cancer treatment (for patients and health professionals), supportive care, screening, and investigational or newly approved drugs. The information is also available in Spanish.

CancerFax also includes more than a hundred fact sheets on various cancer-related topics, selected news items, information on ordering NCI publications, and citations and abstracts on cancer topics extracted monthly from the scientific literature.

To use CancerFax, call the CancerFax computer (301) 402-5874 from the telephone on a fax machine (the machine must be set to touch-tone dialing). After reaching CancerFax, you are asked to select either the English or Spanish version. Then you are told how to obtain the CancerFax contents list of available information and the corresponding six-digit code numbers.

After reviewing the list, call CancerFax again and you will be guided through the steps to select and receive printouts by fax. You request the information you want by entering the appropriate code number into the handset keypad of the fax machine. The faxes you will receive vary considerably in length, from two pages to more than thirty.

CancerFax can be used 24 hours a day, 7 days a week. There is no charge for the service itself. Users pay only for the cost of the telephone call to the CancerFax computer in Maryland.

The American Cancer Society

The American Cancer Society (ACS) is a nationwide, community-based, voluntary health organization dedicated to eliminating cancer as a major health problem by preventing the disease, saving lives from cancer, and diminishing suffering from cancer through research, education and service.

The American Cancer Society has a wide range of programs to assist cancer patients and their families. We briefly describe some of their programs, but they are very happy to talk to you about your individual needs. Their toll-free number is (800) 227-2345, Monday through Friday during regular business hours.

Resources, Information, and Guidance (RIG)

RIG provides the most current information about community and American Cancer Society resources for cancer patients and their families. RIG volunteers act as contact persons for the American Cancer Society and community resources, connecting cancer patients with the available community services, which may include counseling, patient education, support groups, visitation, home care, and patient transportation. The volunteers offer a listening ear for patients' fears and concerns and provide help in finding solutions for the varied problems surrounding your cancer and its treatment.

Cancer Response System

The Cancer Response System is a national toll-free hotline (800-227-2345) you can call Monday through Friday to learn more about a specific type of cancer, its detection, treatment, unproven methods, patient and community services, and the American Cancer Society. This information service is for cancer patients, their friends and family, health professionals, and the general public. When you call the Cancer Response System, trained volunteers or staff will answer your questions and provide you with the most up-to-date information as well as written follow-up materials.

I Can Cope

I Can Cope is a patient and family education program about living with cancer. In a series of classes, doctors, nurses, social workers, other health care professionals and community representatives will provide cancer information and answers to questions about human anatomy, cancer development, diagnosis, treatment, side effects, new research, communication, emotions, sexuality, self-esteem, and community resources.

These free classes provide facts, encouragement, and practical hints through presentations and class discussions to help patients, families, and friends deal with the day-to-day issues of living with cancer.

Look Good . . . Feel Better

The American Cancer Society's Look Good . . . Feel Better program is a community-based, free service teaching female cancer patients beauty techniques to help enhance their appearance and self-image during chemotherapy and radiation treatments. The program is designed to help women recovering from cancer deal with the unpleasant side effects of cancer treatment such as dry skin and loss of hair.

Support Groups

The American Cancer Society has established support groups for sharing experiences, feelings, and coping skills related to cancer. Groups are led by medical professionals or specially trained volunteers who have had cancer.

If you need to talk on a one-on-one basis with someone who has gone through a similar experience, the CanSurmount program is an option. The CanSurmount visitor is a specially trained volunteer who, whenever possible, is matched according to the patient's diagnosis, age, sex, and socioeconomic status.

There is also a one-on-one visitation program for women who have a personal concern about breast cancer. The program provides information and support by someone who has already been through the breast cancer experience herself.

Road to Recovery

Road to Recovery is an American Cancer Society service program providing transportation for cancer patients to their treatments and home again. Sometimes the biggest obstacle to recovery can be getting to and from the treatment center. Volunteer drivers are available in many areas of the United States to help patients overcome this problem. In addition to Road to Recovery, limited financial assistance may be available for long-distance trips to and from treatment.

Home Care Supplies and Special Help

The American Cancer Society has a variety of medical equipment such as hospital beds, walkers, wheelchairs, and other supplies available for loan to cancer patients to allow them to stay comfortably at home while ill or recovering. Insurance and/or Medicare benefits will be utilized when appropriate. Limited financial assistance for services such as housekeeping is available in some areas. Items such as wigs, head scarves, breast prostheses, stoma covers, gowns, slippers, and lap robes are also available in some areas.

Candlelighters

Candlelighters provide information and support on childhood cancer, research, treatment, and community resources. A free quarterly newsletter and youth newsletter are also available. Candlelighters parents' groups meet regularly in several places around the United States.

The American Cancer Society sponsors summer camps for children and teens with cancer. A camp session for siblings of children with cancer is also offered in some states, to help these young people gain a better understanding of the effects of cancer on their lives.

There is also a school reentry program, designed to pave the way for the child who is returning to the classroom after a diagnosis of cancer. A health care professional will provide basic information to the child's classmates regarding the disease and its treatment.

Access to Information Through the Computer

For those people who are "hooked up" to the Internet or the Worldwide Web, a wealth of information is available. We suggest starting at a couple of sites, and "surfing" from there:

CancerNet

CancerNet is probably the most comprehensive and up-to-date source of computerized information about cancer. It is maintained by the National Cancer Institute. It can be reached at *gopher://gopher.nih.gov/11/clin/cancernet*, or send electronic mail to *cancernet@icicb.nci.nih.gov* with no subject, and the word *help* as the message. You will receive back a message explaining how to use the system.

OncoLink

OncoLink is a web and gopher server oriented to cancer, operated by the University of Pennsylvania. This is a very professional-looking resource and is somewhat nicer to use than CancerNet, although you can get to wherever you want to go from either.

- With a web client, such as Netscape or Mosaic, go to *http://oncolink.upenn.edu/*
- With a gopher client go to *gopher oncolink.upenn.edu 80*

Glossary

Accelerator (linear): A machine, often called a linac, that produces high-energy X rays for the treatment of cancer.

Adjuvant therapy: A treatment method used in addition to the primary therapy. Radiation therapy often is used as an adjuvant to surgery or chemotherapy.

Alopecia: Hair loss.

Analgesic: A medication administered to reduce pain.

Anemia: Having too few red blood cells. Symptoms of anemia include feeling tired, weak, and short of breath.

Anorexia: Poor appetite.

Anti-emetic: A drug used to control nausea and vomiting.

Axilla: Armpit area where many lymph nodes are located that drain the arm and breast.

Benign: Describing a slow-growing, not malignant, tumor that does not spread to other parts of the body. If completely removed, benign lesions do not tend to recur. Incompletely removed tumors may recur but will not spread. Although benign, these tumors may cause permanent damage to some structures in the brain.

Bilateral: On both sides of the body.

Biological therapy: Treatment to stimulate or restore the ability of the immune system to fight infection and disease. Also called *immunotherapy*.

Biopsy: The removal of a small portion of a tumor to allow a pathologist to examine it under a microscope and provide a diagnosis of tumor type.

Blood count: The number of red blood cells, white blood cells, and platelets in a sample of blood.

Bone marrow: Spongy tissue in the cavities of large bones, where the body's blood cells are produced.

Brachytherapy: Internal radiation treatment achieved by implanting radioactive material directly into the tumor or very close to it. Sometimes called *internal radiation therapy*.

Cancer: A general name for more than one hundred diseases in which abnormal cells grow out of control; a malignant tumor.

Carcinogenic: A property of some agent (for example, smoke or alcohol) that could contribute to the development of cancer (same as oncogenic).

Carcinoma: The most common type of cancer. It arises from the skin or from the lining of the bowel, bronchus, or duct of a gland, such as in the breast or pancreas.

CAT scan: Computerized axial tomography, often called a *CT scan*, which provides three-dimensional X-ray images of some part of the body. It is useful for diagnosing cancer and for planning radiation therapy treatments.

Catheter: A small, flexible plastic tube inserted into a portion of the body.

CBC: Complete blood count. Determines whether the proper number of red blood cells, white blood cells, and platelets are present in the patient's blood.

Cells: The body is made up of tiny, functioning units called cells.These can be observed under a microscope. Each cell plays a specialized role in the body. Groups of cells are organized together to form tissue. Tissues are organized to form organs in the body.

Central venous catheter: A special thin, flexible tube placed in a large vein. It remains there for as long as it is needed to deliver and withdraw fluids.

Cervix: The lower part of the uterus, which projects out into the vagina.

Chemotherapist: A physician who specializes in the use of drugs to treat cancer; often called a medical oncologist.

Chemotherapy: Treatment with anticancer drugs.

Chromosome: A strand of genes.

Chronic: Persisting for a long time.

Clinical trials: Medical research studies conducted with volunteers. Each study is designed to answer scientific questions and to find better ways to prevent or treat cancer.

CNS: Central nervous system; refers to the brain and spinal cord.

Cobalt 60: A radioactive substance used as a radiation source to treat cancer.

Colon: Large intestine.

Colposcopy: Visual examination of the vagina and cervix through a magnifying instrument inserted into the vagina.

Combination chemotherapy: The use of more than one drug to treat cancer.

Connective tissue: The tissues of the body that bind together and support various structures of the body. Examples are bone, cartilage, and muscle.

Contrast agent: A chemical that is used to highlight disease processes on X-ray tests, contrasting them against the background of normal tissues.

CT-scan (CAT-scan or CT X ray): A three-dimensional X ray. CT stands for computerized tomography.

Cure: An outcome of treatment that leaves the patient disease-free, with no likelihood of recurrence.

Cyst: A cavity, usually filled with a fluid, sometimes associated with benign or malignant tumors.

Dermatitis: A skin rash.

Diagnostic work-up: Performing X-ray and other imaging tests, blood tests, and physical examinations in order to establish a diagnosis.

Dietitian: A professional who plans diet programs for proper nutrition.

Differential diagnosis: A list of the most likely diagnoses for a particular set of symptoms and X-ray findings. The use of different imaging techniques often narrows the differential diagnosis to the most likely disease present.

Diuretics: Drugs that help the body get rid of excess water and salt.

DNA: Abbreviation for deoxyribonucleic acid, the chemical name for the substance making up our genes.

Dosimetrist: A person who plans and calculates the proper radiation dose for treatment.

Dysplasia: Alteration in the size, shape, and organization of cells or tissues.

Edema: Abnormal accumulation of fluid; e.g., pulmonary edema refers to a buildup of fluid in the lungs.

Electron beam: A stream of particles producing high-energy radiation to treat cancer.

Epithelium: A layer of cells in the skin, mucous membrane, or any duct that replaces worn-out cells by cell division.

Excision: Surgical removal.

External radiotherapy: Radiation therapy that uses a machine located outside of the body to aim high-energy rays at cancer cells. Sometimes called external-beam radiotherapy.

Field: A term used in radiation oncology to describe or define an area through which X rays are directed toward the tumor.

Fistula: An abnormal connection between two structures or organs.

Fluoride: A chemical applied to the teeth to prevent tooth decay.

Fluoride therapy: Daily self-application of fluoride gel in a custom-fitted mouthpiece; this may prevent excessive tooth decay after irradiation to the head and neck region.

Fractionation: The daily dose of radiation based on the total dose divided into a particular number of daily treatments.

Frozen section: Technique for rapid microscopic analysis of biopsied tissue.

Gamma rays: High-energy rays coming from a radioactive source such as cobalt 60.

Gastrointestinal: Having to do with the digestive tract, which includes the mouth, esophagus, stomach, and intestines.

GI: gastrointestinal.

Grade: In reference to tumors, the aggressiveness of the cell type, from very low aggressiveness with slow growth pattern to very aggressive with rapid spread. Tumor grading classifications vary according to type of tumor.

Gray: A measurement of radiation dosage.

Gross total resection (GTR): No evidence of residual or remaining tumor on postoperative scans.

Health care professional: Any medical team member involved in patient care, such as a nurse, physician, dietitian, pharmacist, physiotherapist, occupational therapist, social worker, or psychologist.

Hematocrit: The percentage of blood made up of red blood cells.

Hematology: The study of blood and its disorders.

Hemoglobin: The part of red blood cells carrying oxygen to tissues.

High-dose-rate (HDR) remote brachytherapy: A type of internal radiation in which each treatment is given in a few minutes while the radioactive source is in place. The source of radioactivity is removed between treatments. Also known as high-dose-rate remote radiation therapy.

Hormones: Natural substances released by an organ that can influence the function of other organs in the body.

Hyperfractionated radiation: Division of the total dose of radiation into smaller doses given more than once a day.

Hyperthermia: The elevation of tissue temperature; a cancer treatment known to enhance the curative effects of irradiation and chemotherapy.

Hypopharynx: Part of the lower throat beside and behind the larynx (or voice box).

Immune system: The body's defense system that protects it from foreign substances such as bacteria and viruses that are harmful to the body.

Implant: A quantity of radioactive material placed in or near a cancer.

Increased intracranial pressure: Increased pressure within the brain.

Infusion: Slow and/or prolonged intravenous delivery of a drug or fluids.

Internal radiation: A type of therapy in which a radioactive substance is implanted into or close to the area needing treatment. Usually termed *brachytherapy*.

Interstitial implant: The placement of fine tubes in a gridlike pattern through tissues containing a cancer; these tubes are filled later with radioactive sources for brachytherapy.

Interstitial radiation: A radioactive source (implant) placed directly into the tissue (not in a body cavity).

Intracavitary implant: The placement of a small tube within a body cavity, such as the bronchus or vagina; this tube is later filled with radioactive sources for brachytherapy.

Intracavitary radiation: A radioactive source (implant) placed in a body cavity such as the chest cavity or the vagina.

Intraoperative radiation: A type of external radiation used to deliver a large dose of radiation therapy to the tumor bed and surrounding tissue at the time of surgery.

Intravenous (IV): Into a vein.

Ionizing radiation: A type of radiation used in cancer treatment that damages DNA and stops cell growth. Examples include X rays, gamma rays, electrons, and neutrons.

Ipsilateral: On the same side of the body (opposite of contralateral).

Isotope: A radioactive substance used in diagnosis or treatment of cancer.

Karnofsky score: A measure of the patient's overall physical health following treatment, judged by his or her level of activity.

Larynx: Part of the throat used for speaking; often called the *voice box* or *Adam's apple.*

Layperson: One not trained in professional (medical) matters.

Leukemia: A malignant cancer of the blood-forming tissues (bone marrow or lymph nodes), generally characterized by an overproduction of white blood cells.

Leukocyte: White blood cell.

Linear accelerator: A machine creating high-energy radiation to treat cancers, using electricity to form a stream of fast-moving subatomic particles. Also called megavoltage linear accelerator or a linac.

Local invasion: The spread of cancer from an original site to the surrounding tissues.

Localized tumors: Tumors that are contained in one particular site and have not yet spread.

Lymph node: A collection of lymphocytes within a capsule and connected to other lymph nodes by fine lymphatic vessels; a common site for certain cancer cells to grow after traveling along lymphatic vessels.

Lymphatic system: A network of fine lymphatic vessels that collect tissue fluids from all over the body and return these fluids to the blood. Accumulations of lymphocytes, called lymph nodes, are situated along the course of lymphatic vessels.

Lymphocyte: A type of white blood cell that helps protect the body against invading organisms by producing antibodies and regulating the immune system response.

Lymphoma: A type of cancer beginning in an altered lymphocyte. There are two broad categories of lymphomas, Hodgkin's disease and non-Hodgkin's lymphoma. Both respond favorably to radiation and chemotherapy drugs.

Macrophage: A type of white blood cell assisting in the body's fight against bacteria and infection by engulfing and destroying invading organisms.

Malignant: Tending to grow quickly and spread, causing harm to surrounding and/or distant tissue.

Mammogram: An X ray of the breast used to detect cancer, sometimes before it can be detected by palpation. Women over fifty are advised to have a mammogram every year; women in their forties every two years.

Medical oncologist: A doctor specializing in using chemotherapy to treat cancer.

Medical physicist: A physicist with specialized training for determining how to use radiation as safely as possible. Sometimes called a radiation physicist.

Melanoma: A type of cancer that begins in the pigment-containing cells of a skin mole or the lining of the eye.

Meningioma: A type of brain tumor that is relatively common and usually benign.

Menopause: The time in a woman's life when ovarian function diminishes and menstrual cycles stop, usually at forty-five to fifty years of age.

Metastases: When cancer cells break away from their original site and spread to other parts of the body.

Metastatic cancer: An advanced stage of cancer in which cells from the original (primary) site have spread (metastasized) to other organs.

Morbidity: Sickness, side effects, and symptoms of a treatment or disease.

MRI (magnetic resonance imaging): A method of taking pictures of body tissue using magnetic fields.

Mucositis: Inflammation of the lining of areas such as the mouth.

Nasopharynx: Part of the breathing passage behind the nasal cavity.

Neurologist: A physician specializing in nonsurgical diseases of the nervous system.

Neurology: The study of the nervous system and its diseases.

Neuro-oncologist: A physician specializing in the treatment of tumors of the nervous system.

Neurosurgeon: A physician specializing in surgery of the nervous system.

Oncogenic: A factor or agent with the potential to cause cancer (same as carcinogenic).

Oncologist: A physician specializing in the study and treatment of cancer.

Oncology: The study of cancer.

Palliative care: Treatment to relieve, rather than cure, symptoms caused by cancer. Palliative care can help people live more comfortably.

Palpate: To examine by carefully feeling with the fingers.

Pathologist: A specialist who attempts to describe the nature of a disease by analyzing samples obtained from tissues, organs, or body fluids. Samples or biopsy specimens of brain tumors, for example, are surgically obtained by the neurosurgeon. Analysis of a brain biopsy is a tedious procedure. A final report from the pathologist may not be available for three or more days. It is the pathologist who carefully analyzes the specimen and makes a judgment on the diagnosis.

Pathology: The study of diseased tissues, both by gross and by microscopic examination, of tissues removed during surgery or postmortem. The pathologist is a physician with specialized training in performing and interpreting these examinations.

Pharynx: Medical term for the throat from the nasal and oral cavities above to the larynx and esophagus below.

Physical therapist: A health professional trained in the use of treatments such as exercise and massage.

Platelets: Special blood cells that help stop bleeding.

Portal film: An X-ray film of the anatomic area designated to be treated with radiation.

Primary tumor: The place where the cancer originates, which is referred to regardless of the site of its eventual spread. Thus, prostate cancer that spreads to the bone is still prostate cancer, and is not referred to as bone cancer.

Prognosis: The predicted or likely outcome.

Prophylactic: Preventive measure or medication.

Prostate: A gland at the base of the bladder in males for the production of seminal fluids. Cancer of this gland is common in elderly men.

Protocol: A standardized combination of therapies developed specifically for particular tumors.

Proton: A positively charged particle found in every atomic nucleus.

Radiation: Energy carried by waves or a stream of particles.

Radiation dose: The amount of radiation absorbed by an irradiated object. This dose is recorded in Gray (Gy).

Radiation dosimetrist: A specialized radiation technologist who calculates the exact amount of radiation to be given to a radiation therapy patient each day. Some dosimetrists also manufacture customized blocks to shield normal tissues and/or support devices to help patients hold still during therapy.

Radiation oncologist: A physician specializing in the treatment of tumors by radiation therapy.

Radiation physicist: A person trained to ensure the radiation machine delivers the right amount of radiation to the treatment site.

Radiation portal (radiation field): The area under treatment with radiation.

Radiation therapist: A person with special training who runs the equipment that delivers the radiation. Sometimes called a radiation technologist.

Radiation therapy: The use of radiation to treat disease.

Radiation therapy nurse: A nurse with extra training in the support and care of patients receiving radiation therapy.

Radiation therapy technologist: A technician trained to accurately deliver the doses of radiation prescribed by the radiation oncologist, under the supervision of radiation physicists and radiation oncologists. Also known as a radiation therapist.

Radioactivity: A property of all unstable elements that regularly change (or "decay") to an altered state by releasing energy in the form of photons (gamma rays) or particles (electrons, alpha particles, etc.).

Radiologist: A physician with special training in reading diagnostic X rays and performing specialized X-ray procedures.

Radiotherapy: Radiation therapy.

Recurrence: The return of a cancer after all detectable traces had been removed by primary therapy; recurrences may be local (near the primary site) or distant (metastatic).

Regional involvement: The spread of cancer to areas near the original site and not to distant areas of the body.

Relapse: Recurrence of the disease following treatment.

Remission, complete: Condition in which no cancerous cells can be detected by a microscope, and the patient appears to be free of disease.

Remission, partial: Generally means that by all methods used to measure the existence of a tumor, there has been at least a 50 percent regression of the disease following treatment.

Remote brachytherapy: See high-dose-rate remote brachy-therapy.

Resection: Surgical removal; in relation to cancer resection, the pathologist often indicates if the outer margins of the resection had no cancer cells present or were "negative."

Sarcoma: A type of cancer derived from connective bone or fat tissues. Examples include fibrosarcoma, osteogenic sarcoma, and liposarcoma.

Scan: A diagnostic test usually involving the movement or scanning of a detector to produce a picture. Examples include ultrasound, nuclear medicine scan, computer-assisted tomography (CAT), or magnetic resonance imaging (MRI) scans.

Secondary cancer: Cancer arising from a primary cancer; metastatic cancer.

Side effects: Symptoms directly related to treatment, such as the side effect of nausea resulting from radiation treatment over the stomach. Side effects are considered *acute* when they occur during treatment and subside when treatment is complete. Those symptoms persisting over a longer period of time are considered *chronic*.

Simulation: A process involving special X-ray pictures used to plan radiation treatment so that the area to be treated is precisely located and marked for treatment.

Site: The location of the tumor.

Solid tumor: A cancer originating in an organ or tissue other than bone marrow or the lymph system.

Stage: The anatomic extent of the cancer. Cancer may exist in the organ of origin, extend locally, or spread to regional tissues, then to local lymph nodes, and then to distant areas as metastases.

Stomatitis: Sores on the inside lining of the mouth.

Subtotal resection: Removal of the majority, but not all of a tumor.

Systemic: Having a widespread effect on the body as a whole, rather than just local tissue.

TBI: Total body irradiation.

Treatment port or field: The place on the body at which the radiation beam is aimed.

Tumor: An abnormal growth of cells or tissues. Tumors may be benign (noncancerous) or malignant (cancerous).

Ultrasound: A technique for taking a picture of internal organs or other structures using sound waves.

White blood cells: The blood cells that fight infection.

Xerostomia: Dryness of the mouth caused by malfunctioning salivary glands.

X ray: Radiation used at low levels to diagnose disease, or at high levels to treat cancer.

Index

Page numbers in **boldface** indicate either illustrations or tables in the text.

adjuvant treatment, 29–30
  for breast cancer, 61, 67
  hormones, 41–42
afterloader technique, 33–34, 126,
  128–129
aggressiveness of tumor. *See* grade
  of tumor
alkylating agents, 39
American Board of Medical
  Physics, 49
American Board of Radiology, 47,
  48, 49
American Cancer Society, 15–16
  resources, 173, 175–179
American Registry of Radiologic
  Technologists, 49
American Society of Radiation
  Technologists, 50
anticancer drugs, 39–41
  administration methods, 40
antimetabolic drugs, 39
appetite loss, 134–135
astrocytomas, 105, 106–107, 177

Bell, Alexander Graham, 125
benign tumors, 4, 22
biopsies, 20–21, 111, 138
  CT-guided, 21, 91, 98
  excisional, 21
  incisional, 21

blood, cancer of. *See* leukemia
bone marrow transplantation, 59,
  68–69
books, 171–173
boron neutron capture therapy
  (BNCT), 38–39
brachytherapy. *See* internal radiotherapy
brain, 103, **103**
  irradiation of, 89–90
brain cancer treatment options,
  106–109
  for astrocytomas, 106–107
  chemotherapy, 107
  for meningiomas, 107–108
  for metastases, 108–109
  radiotherapy, 106–107, 108
  surgery, 106–107, 108
  watch-and-wait option, 106
brain tumors, 102–109
  benign, 104
  BNCT for, 38–39
  debulking, 43
  malignant, 104
  metastatic, 102–103, 104–105,
    108–109
  primary, 102
  radiosurgery for, 33–34
  small-cell lung cancer and, 89–90
  symptoms, 104

brain tumors (*continued*)
  types of, 104–106
breast, female, 54
  lymph nodes near, **54**, 55
breast cancer
  ductal carcinoma *in situ*, 55, 65
  estrogen-receptor status and, 58
  heredity and, 7
  infiltrating lobular cancer, 56
  invasive, 55–56
  lymph nodes and, **54**, 55, **57**,
    58, 60
  mammograms for detection
    of, 15
  metastases, **57**, 58
  noninvasive, 55
  outlook, 56, 69
  progesterone-receptor status
    and, 58
  types of, 55–56
breast cancer treatment options,
    59–69
  breast-conserving, 59–60, 63–65,
    140, 143, 151–152
  for DCIS-66, 65
  doctors, attitudes and,139–140
  hospital size and, 143
  for lobular carcinoma *in situ*, 66
  lumpectomy and radiotherapy,
    59–60, 63–65, **139**, 140, 143,
    151–152
  lumpectomy/chemotherapy/
    radiotherapy, 59–60, 62
  mastectomy, 60
  non–breast-conserving, 59, 60,
    61, 63–65, 140
  radiotherapy, 60–61, 62, 64–65,
    67, 68
  stage of cancer and, 62, 65–69
  surgery, 42–43
  tainoxifen, 42
bronchoscopy, 19

CancerFax, 174–175
Cancer Information Service, 174
CancerNet, 179
cancers. *See also* specific cancers
  diagnosis of, 15–26
  factors in development of, 6–8
  as generic term, 1
  heredity and, 7
  Comprehensive Cancer Centers,
    142, 161–166
  considerations in choosing,
    140–141, 144–145
carcinoma, defined, 5
cell division
  of cancerous cells, 2, 4
  DNA and, 1–2
  healthy, control of by DNA, 1–2
  tumor formation and, 2, 3
Centers of Excellence, 141, 142–143
cervical cancer, 90–98
  detection of, 90–91
  Pap smear test for, 15, 20, 90, 91
  stages of, 92
  TNM system for classifying, 92
cervical cancer treatment options
  fertility and, 95, 96
  intracavitary brachytherapy, 33
  radiotherapy, 92, 93, 94, **94**,
    97, 98
  stage of cancer and, 95–98
cervix, 91, **91**
chemotherapy, 29, 30, 39–41
  for brain cancers, 107
  for breast cancer, 61–63
  for cervical cancer, 97, 98
  defined, 39
  duration of treatment, 40–41, 62
  medical oncologists and, 139
  for non-small-cell lung cancer,
    88, 89
  side effects, 41
  use of, 39, 40

Clinical Cancer Centers,
    NCI-designated, 141–142,
    167–169
CMF, 40
cobalt machines, 31, 123
collimators, 122, 123
colon cancer, heredity and, 7
colonoscopy, 19
combination treatment, 29
Comprehensive Cancer Centers,
    NCI-designated, 141–142, 161–166
computer access to information,
    179
computerized tomography. See CT
conization, 95
Crick, Francis, 2
cryosurgery, 95
CT (computerized tomography),
    17, 121
    guided biopsies, 21
curative treatments, 44–45
cure, realistic chances of, 27
Curie, Pierre, 14
cytological studies, 20

debulking, 43
dental decay, 133
diagnosis of cancer, 15–26
    early, importance of,15
    facing, 26–27
    initial suspicion, 15–16
    warninq signals, 15–16
diagnostic tests
    of grade of tumor, 22–23
    imaging tests, 16–20
    tissue sample examination, 20–21
diarrhea, 132–133
diathermy, 95
diet, 132
dietitian, 51, 125
DNA, 1–2, 3
    effect of radiation on, 10–11

dosimetrist, 50, 122
double helix, 2, 3
drugs, anticancer, 39–41
dry mouth, 133, 134

endometrial cancer, 98–102
    stages and grades, 99, 99
    symptoms, 98
endometrial cancer treatment
    options, 100–102
    fertility and, 100
    radiotherapy, 99–100, 101,
        102, 127
    surgery, 99–101
endometrium, 98
endoscopy, 19–20
engineers, 123
estrogen-receptor status, 58
external radiotherapy, 31–32, 74,
    93, 117
    daily treatments, 122–125
    as painless, 119, 124
    simulation process, 119–122, 120
    technique, 31,32
    X rays and, 9–10, 32
eye tumors, proton radiotherapy
    for, 38

fatigue, as side effect, 131
fax, information by, 174–175
fertility, radiotherapy and, 14
follow-up care, 135

gamma knife, 34, 35, 109
gamma rays, 10, 32, 33
glioma, defined, 5
glottic cancer, 111, 112, 113–114
glottis, 110
grade of tumor
    breast tumor cells, 58
    defined, 22
    histological grade, 23

grade of tumor (*continued*)
  nuclear grade, 22
  treatment options and, 23

hairloss, 133
head and neck cancers, 109–117.
    See also laryngeal cancer;
    oral cancers
health maintenance organizations
    (HMOS), 146
healthy cells, effects of radiation
    on, 12
heredity
  and cancers, 7
  radiotherapy and, 13–14
high-dose-rate, 93, 128
hormone suppression therapy, for
    prostate cancer, 77–78, 83
hormone therapy, 41–42, 100
for breast cancer, 58, 61–63, 67
hospitals, choosing
  large vs. small, 143
  teaching hospitals, 142–143
hyperthermia, 37
hysterectomy, 95, 96, 99–100

imaging tests,16–20
  direct, 19–20
  indirect, 16–19
incontinence, prostatectomy and, 77
information resources, 171–179
insurance,medical, 146
internal radiotherapy, 33–34, 74,
    93, **94**, 117
  and external radiotherapy,
    125–126
  gamma rays and, 10, 32, 33
  high-dose-rate, 93,128
  interstitial, 33–34, 128–130, **129**
  intracavitary, 33, 126–128, **127**
Internet resources, 179

interstitial internal radiotherapy,
    33–34, 128–130, **129**
intracavitary internal radiotherapy,
    33, 126–128, 127
intraoperative radiotherapy, 37–38
ionization, 10

larynx, 110, **110**
laryngeal cancer, 109–114
  stages of, 111, 111–114
  symptoms, 110–111
laryngeal cancer treatment options,
    111–115
  side–effects, 111–112
leukemia, defined, 5
LHRH agonist drugs, 77–78
linear accelerators, 31, 32, 123
lip cancers, 116–117
lobectomy, 85
lumpectomy, 59–60, 61
lung cancer, 83–85
  pollution and 7
  stage groupings, 24, **26**, 85
  and superior vena cava
    syndrome, 89
  TNM system for classifying, 24,
    25, 85, **86**
lung cancer, non-small-cell, 84, 85
  treatment options, 85–89
lung cancer, small-cell, 84–85,
    89–90
  treatment options, 89–90
lungs, 83–84, **84**
Lupron, 77
lymph nodes, 6
  biopsies of, 21
  breast, **54**, 55
  and breast cancer, **54**, 55, **57**,
    58, 60
  cancer in, and stage of tumor, 23
  near lungs, **84**, 87, 88

removal of, 43
lymphoma, defined, 5

magnetic resonance imaging. *See* MRI
malignant tumors, 4, 22. *See* cancers
  appearance of cells, 22
mammograms, 15
managed care, 146
mastectomy, 60, 66, 67
medical oncologists, 138
medical physicist, 48–49, 122
meningiomas, 105, 107–108
metastases, 22
  brain, 102–103
  defined, 5
  distant or extensive, and stage of cancer, 23–24, 45
  methods of, 5–6
microwaves, 37
misoprostol, 37
modified radical mastectomy, 60
  sexual potency and, 75, 77, 78, 81, 83
  stage of cancer and, 79, 80–83
  surgery, 73, 76–77, 79, 80, 81, 82, 83
  watch-and-wait option, 72, 73, 78–79
prostatectomy, 76–77, 80,81
prostate gland, 69,70
proton radiotherapy, 38
PSA (prostate-specific antigen) test, 15, 20, 70–71

quality of life, 152–153

radiation
  as cause of cancer, 12–13
  genetic effects of, 13–14
  types of, 9–10

radiation oncologists, 47–48, 120, 122, 138
  board-certification, 145
  choosing, 47–48, 140
  communicating with, 149–150
  considerations in choosing, 145–147
  importance of seeing, 139
radiation therapists, 49–50, 121
radiation therapy. *See* radiotherapy
radiation therapy nurses, 50–51
radiation therapy technologists, 49–50, 120, 123
radical mastectomy, 60, 67–68
radical prostatectomy, 76–77, 80, 81
radioactive seeds, 33–34
radioactivity, 119, 126, 127–128, 129, 130
radio frequency waves, 37
radioimmunotherapy (RIT), 36–37
radiolabeled antibody therapy, 36–37
radioprotectors, 37
radiosensitizers, 37
radiosurgery,34–35, 108
radiotherapy, 29–39,
  See also external radiotherapy; internal radiotherapy
  advantages and disadvantages, 151–152
  basic rule of, 30
  for brain cancers, 106–107, 108
  for breast cancer, 60–61
  for cervical cancer, 92, 93, 94, 94, 96, 97, 98
  defined, 30
  effects on healthy tissue,12
  for endometrial cancer, 99–100, 101, 102
  external, 31–32
  fears about, 151–152

radiotherapy (*continued*)
  goal, 30
  for head and neck cancers, 109
  for laryngeal cancers, 111–114
  major developments, 14–15
  new types of, 34–39
  for non-small-cell lung cancer, 87,
    88, 89
  for oral cancers, 114–117
  palliative, 30–31, 37
  for prostate cancer,74–75
  side effects, 12, 130–136,
    151, 152
  versus surgery, 151
  treatment decisions regarding,
    137–154
  treatment steps, 119–130
radiotherapy machine, **121**
radiotherapy team, 47–52, 120,
  124, 129
radiotherapy treatment centers, 144
recurrence of cancer, signs of, 136
remote afterloader. *See* afterloader
  technique
Roentgen, Wilhelm, 9, 14

salagen, 134
salivary gland tumors, 38
sarcoma, defined, 5
secondary tumors, 22
sexual potency
  and hormone suppression
    therapy, 77–78, 83
  and prostate cancer radio-
    therapy, 75
  and prostate cancer surgery,
    76–77
  prostate cancer treatment options
    and, 75, 76, 77, 78, 81, 83
  watch-and-wait option and, 81
sexual problems
  cervical cancer treatment and, 97

side effects
  of chemotherapy, 41
  of hormone therapy, 42
  of radiotherapy, 12, 130–136,
    151, 152
simulation process, 119–122, **120**
size of tumor
  breast conservation and, 68
  stage of cancer and, 23
skin care, 136
skin soreness, 131–132
social workers, 51
stage of cancer. *See also* TNM system
  breast cancer, 56, **57**, 62
  factors determining, 23–24
  lung cancer, 24, **26**
  treatment options and, 23
  various types of tumors in
    relation to, 24
subglottis, 110
superior vena cava syndrome, 89
support, psychological, 123,
  147–149
support groups, 52, 148–149
supraglottic cancer, 111, 112,
  113–114
supraglottis, 110
surgery, 29,30, 42–44
  for brain cancers, 106–107, 108
  breast-conserving, 43
  for cervical cancer, 95, 96–97
  definitive, aim of, 43–44
  for endometrial cancer, 99–101
  exploratory, 20–21
  intraoperative radiotherapy and,
    37–38
  for laryngeal cancers, 111–114
  for non-small-cell lung cancer,
    85, 87–88, 89
  for oral cancers, 114, 116, 117
  for prostate cancer, 76–77, 79, 80,
    81, 82, 83

reconstructive, 43, 44
surgical oncologists and, 139
types of, 43–44
surgical oncologists, 138, 139
Systemic treatment, 39–41, 61–62

tamoxifen, 42, 63
teaching hospitals, 142–143
tests for cancer. *See* diagnostic tests
three-dimensional conformal radio-
    therapy, 35–36, **36**, 74
tiredness, as side effect, 131
tissue sample examination, 20–21
TNM system
    for classifying lung cancer, 24, **25**
    for describing breast cancers, 56,
        57, 68
    for describing cervical cancer,
        92, **92**
    for describing laryngeal cancers,
        111, **111**
    factors comprising, 24, 56
tongue cancers, 115–116
treatment decisions, 137–154
    quality of life and, 153
    step-by-step approach to making,
        153–154
treatment options, 29–45. *See also*
    specific cancers and types
    of treatment
    chemotherapy, 29, 39–41
    choosing, 26

doctors' attitudes and, 139–140
grade of tumor and, 23
hormone therapy, 41–42
managed care and, 146
multitechnique, 29–30
radiotherapy, 29–39
realistic, 27
stage of cancer and, 23
surgery, 29, 30, 42–44
weighing odds, 150–152
tumors
    benign, 4
    malignant, 4
    malignant (*see also* cancers)
    out-of-control cell division
        and, 2, **4**
ultrasound, 18–19, 37
unresectable tumors, 43–44

vaginal cancer, intracavitary
    brachytherapy for, 33
videos, 173
vocal cords, 110, 111, 112, 113

warning signals of cancer, 15–16
Watson, James, 2

X rays, 32, 121, 125
    defined, 9
    as diagnostic tool, 17
    effect on DNA, 10–11
    energy of, 10